Just Add Nature

Rebecca Frank

Just Add Nature

How to boost your
health and happiness,
wherever you live

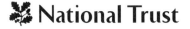
National Trust

Published by National Trust Books

An imprint of HarperCollins Publishers,
1 London Bridge Street, London SE1 9GF
www.harpercollins.co.uk

HarperCollins Publishers, Macken House,
39/40 Mayor Street Upper, Dublin 1, D01 C9W8, Ireland

First published 2024

© National Trust Books 2024
Text © Rebecca Frank
Illustrations © Claire Harrup

ISBN 978-0-00-864136-8

10 9 8 7 6 5 4 3 2 1

The contents of this publication are believed correct at the time of printing.
Nevertheless, the publisher can accept no responsibility for errors or omissions,
changes in the detail given or for any expense or loss thereby caused.

A catalogue record for this book is available from the British Library.
Printed and bound in India.

If you would like to comment on any aspect of this book, please contact us at the
above address or national.trust@harpercollins.co.uk

National Trust publications are available at National Trust shops or online at
nationaltrustbooks.co.uk

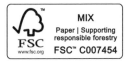

This book is produced from independently certified FSC™ paper
to ensure responsible forest management.

For more information visit: www.harpercollins.co.uk/green

Contents

Introduction

Humans have lived in close contact with nature for most of our history. We evolved to exist in a diverse and natural environment. Yet, increasingly, we immerse ourselves in a life spent indoors, plugged in and shut off from the outside world. And what happens when humans disconnect from nature? We both suffer.

There is now an abundance of scientific evidence that exposure to nature is linked with improved physiological and psychological health. Study after study has shown how nature benefits us physically, emotionally, socially and spiritually. Nature is both a vitamin and a painkiller, a prevention and cure. It is good for us in the moment and serves us well in the long term.

While any time spent in nature is beneficial, the evidence suggests that it is when we truly engage and connect with nature that the real magic happens. You can walk through an ancient woodland with headphones on, looking down at your phone with your mind on an impending deadline, and it will be a very different experience from one where you look up, slow down, switch on your senses and immerse yourself in your surroundings. When we connect with nature and feel a

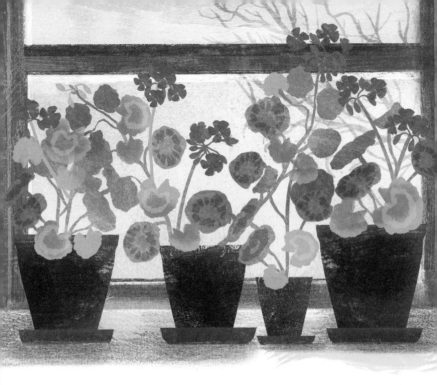

part of it, rather than being just an observer, it alters our brain chemistry and affects how we think, feel and behave.

Of course, nature means very different things to different people, so we need to find ways to access and connect with nature that align with where we live, our passions and our interests. Then we will realise that it needn't require a lot of time or effort to introduce more nature into our lives. It might be walking the greener route to work, buying a couple of houseplants for your home or office or some vegetable seeds to grow on a windowsill, starting a nature journal or spending a night camping under the stars. There are many, many ways to connect with nature, appreciate its beauty and feel a part of the natural world. They aren't necessarily new ideas, but they're more important now than ever.

Spending time in nature should not be a luxury or even a nice-to-have. It's a must-have for all, regardless of age, gender, ethnicity or background. As more of us live in cities we need to find ways to make our urban areas greener and motivate people of all ages to spend more time outdoors, explore and reconnect with the nature on their doorstep. As the evidence mounts, experts are starting to quantify what nature connection can do for our health, and how getting people outside more often can translate to reduced healthcare expenditure. We're seeing green social prescribing, which enables healthcare professionals to recommend nature-based activities as part of a care package to improve mental health. New nature tech can measure our nature deficit and encourage us to get outside for our daily dose of the natural world. 'Motivating people to get outdoors is proving to be one of the most impactful behaviour interventions that exist, and it's relatively cost free, with no

> *Spending time in nature should not be a luxury or even a nice-to-have.*

side effects,' says Jared Hanley of NatureQuant, a US-based company that develops technology to assess and promote nature exposure.

There's no doubt that these are challenging times for humans and for our planet, but it's not too late to help each other. When we engage more with nature, we start to think more consciously about the environment and what we can do to protect it. Eco-anxiety is a real issue for many, but connecting with nature and channelling those feelings into positive action happens to be the best cure for humans and for nature.

Use this book as an invitation to embrace the abundance, beauty and complexity of nature. A reminder to look outside the human world and connect with wildness in the many ways that are available to us. For inspiration to play, work, rest and create using nature as your healer and your guide. And as a call to action to become part of a collective that protects our wild spaces.

Because nature needs you – and you need nature.

*'The world is big and I want to have
a good look at it before it gets dark.'*

John Muir, author and naturalist

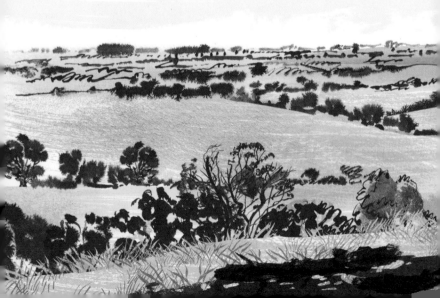

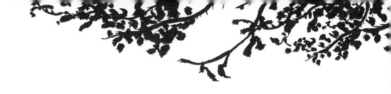

Chapter One

Getting Closer
to Nature

To reconnect with nature, it helps to remind ourselves how entangled with nature we already are. It can be easy to forget, when many of us spend much of our time in houses, cars, offices and gyms, that we exist because of and in conjunction with the natural world. We walk beneath the trees that give us the oxygen we breathe, yet barely notice these incredible species towering above us.

Research shows that the more time we spend in natural environments, the closer and more connected to nature we feel and the more our attention shifts from ourselves to the outside world. People who live and work close to the land could no more imagine a life deprived of nature than some of us could bear the thought of living without our smartphone. Biophilia, a term that literally translates to 'love of life', refers to the theory that humans are genetically drawn to nature and non-human life forms. Edward O. Wilson, a Harvard biologist, first explored the hypothesis in his 1984 book *Biophilia*, where he examined theories to support this innate need for nature, linking back to evolution. It is why we're instinctively drawn to natural environments that were once essential to our survival (water, vegetation, wildlife); it is also the reason we can't resist stopping to take pictures of newborn lambs or the first flowers to emerge after winter, constantly awestruck by the cycle of nature.

Nature has always been necessary to humans as a means of survival. Even today, when most of us no longer need to be closely connected to the land for day-to-day sustenance, this can leave us lacking in the more subtle yet powerful benefits of a relationship with nature. This 'nature deficit' has a wide impact on our health, from increased obesity to decreased attention and a greater risk of physical and mental illness.

Getting closer to nature in ways that align with our lives and our interests will help to reignite our evolutionary pull towards the natural world. If we can learn the names of some of the creatures we live alongside, or grow one item of food rather than buying it pre-packaged from a supermarket, for example, it will increase our connection with nature as well as reducing environmental impact.

The symbiotic relationship that enables species to survive and thrive is needed more than ever in our modern world. As American naturalist Henry David Thoreau wrote in 1851, in the opening of his renowned essay, *Walking*: 'I wish to speak a word on nature, for absolute freedom and wildness, as contrasted with a freedom and culture merely civil – to regard man as an inhabitant, or a part and parcel of Nature, rather than a member of society.' Thoreau's fear that we would one day lose our 'wild and dusky knowledge' in favour of 'lettered learning' has become a real threat, and time is of the essence if we want to recover what has been lost or damaged.

More recently, in her book *Losing Eden*, author Lucy Jones wrote: 'If we continue to take the path of detachment and divorce from nature, at a time of growing biodiversity loss and catastrophic global warming, the consequences of our eco-illiteracy will grow even more hazardous. Nature isn't just beautiful and intriguing, it's our life support system.'

It's clear that if we spend a little time getting to know the natural world that surrounds us better, teach our children and grandchildren about our relationship to plants and wildlife, and let them experience the mood-boosting effect of a romp through the woods or an evening spent gazing at the stars, we will inevitably see that connection deepen. And from that place, nature can work its magic.

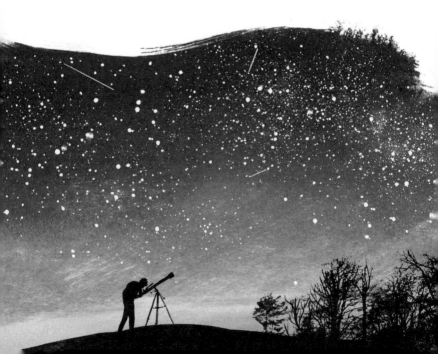

The joy of noticing

When we stop to consciously observe wildlife, we can find ourselves overcome with feelings of awe. You might experience this while seeing giraffes in a safari park or watching a robin visiting a bird feeder outside the kitchen window. The point isn't whether you've spotted one of the 'Big Five'; it's what you've noticed and how much attention you've given it. Most of us don't really pay much attention to the wildlife on our doorstep and yet, if we can become more attuned to the creatures around us, noticing their habits and spotting the species that appear at different times of the day and year, it will bring about a new relationship with nature and change how we perceive our position in the natural world.

Consider how each unique creature plays its role, all interconnected in the vast network of life. Imagine the world from their perspective as they swoop between trees, land on the petals of a flower or scurry through the leaf litter. Does it make your own little world seem suddenly small and strange? Studies at the University of California, Irvine, showed that experiencing awe in nature encourages pro-environmental and pro-social behaviours, so we act more considerately and generously towards the environment and society in ways such as sharing, donating and volunteering.

Looking up

Many of us are guilty of walking around with our heads down, looking at our phones or the ground in front of us. When we look up as we walk, our eyes instantly start to scan the landscape around us and we engage optic flow, which provides us with a panoramic view of motion in our surroundings. Optic flow is enabled by cells in the back of the retina that trigger our system of balance and, according to research by Stanford neuroscientist Dr Andrew Huberman, make us feel calmer by quietening the amygdala – the centre for emotional response in the brain. This link between the cells in the retina and our emotional centre and memory form the basis of EMDR (Eye Movement Desensitisation and Reprocessing), a form of trauma therapy that uses eye movement to help treat people with Post Traumatic Stress Disorder (PTSD). The therapy was first developed by Dr Francine Shapiro who noticed that while walking and scanning the landscape in her local park she felt calmer and less anxious. Panoramic vision can be a great antidote to long hours working on a computer, which involves intense focal vision.

Hunting for nature clues

Once you start looking more closely, you'll soon notice things that you might have overlooked before. Spotting subtle signs of growth, life and movement can give a walk a new focus and enhance your feelings of connection with the natural world. Tristan Gooley, aka The Natural Navigator, is passionate about the benefits of using our eyes and ears as natural navigation tools (as opposed to maps and apps). Looking at the shape of a tree canopy, for example, can help you to work out which side of the tree gets the most sun and wind exposure, and therefore which direction you are facing. In countries in northern latitudes the sun spends most of its time in the southern part of the sky, so a thicker, denser canopy on one side of a tree will usually indicate that it is south-facing. In the UK, the prevailing wind is from the south-west so the tops of exposed trees will often lean from south-west to north-east. In cities, algae will thrive on the northern, shadier side of a building and spiders' webs are found on the sheltered side of trees, fences and buildings. Animal behaviour can predict weather changes, and searching for tracks through footprints, feathers, fur and faeces provides an entertaining focus on a walk for both children and grown-ups. Leaves can provide clues

Leaves can provide clues about creatures that share the same habitat.

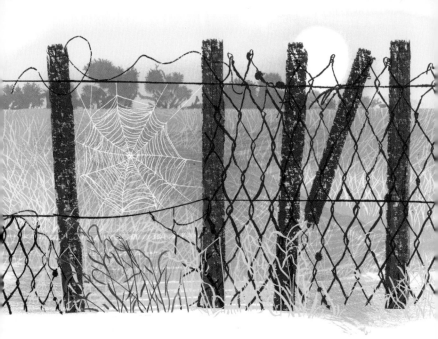

about creatures that share the same habitat, for example, and a change in grasses will indicate when you're close to a river. The appearance of nettles will suggest that you're approaching a village; this fascinating indicator may even offer clues to ancient settlements and is due to the phosphate and nitrate-rich soil in which nettles flourish – often a result of the way the land was farmed by our ancestors, as well as the presence of human refuse, ash and bones.

Putting a name to it

As you become more observant and interested in your surroundings, you'll naturally want to learn about the things that you see. Birds, flowers, trees and butterflies all acquire new meaning when you're able to recognise and name some of the different species and unique characteristics. If something grabs your attention, take a picture or make a note and do some investigation – borrow a field guide, download an app, use Google or ask questions when you're with people who know about your subject. You could contribute your findings to help with different research projects – citizen or community science volunteers play an important role in gathering the enormous amount of data required by scientists and environmentalists and don't usually need any specific skills or qualifications. You could be spotting local wildlife or monitoring plants to help build up a picture of what is present and what might be declining. It's a great way to learn more about a specific field and feel that you're contributing to the conservation of your area. The National Plant Monitoring Scheme (NPMS) is a project where people volunteer to identify and monitor plant species in 1 square kilometre (⅓ square mile) of land close to where they

If something grabs your attention, take a picture or make a note and do some investigation.

live, helping to gather data on plant populations throughout the country. Visit npms.org.uk to see available squares in your area and once signed up you'll be sent information on the different indicator species for your habitat.

If you're prone to overthinking or anxiety, having something to gently distract your mind while you're outdoors can help to quell the dreaded rumination that can surface when alone with your thoughts. 'Getting outdoors to obsess about nature was crucial to my staying sane,' writes journalist Isabel Hardman in her book *The Natural Health Service*. A fixation with plants helps Hardman to refocus her mind when overwhelmed with fear. Be careful not to let a fascination with spotting and naming things get in the way of appreciating simple beauty though – if you're already a keen spotter, sometimes going out without any intention of finding things can make you see your surroundings in a different way.

Getting your hands dirty

Gardeners know that there's much more to gardening than having a pretty space in which to relax. Much like the runner's high there is the gardener's glow, caused largely by direct contact with the serotonin-boosting microbes found in the soil. A garden holds many of the tools we need to boost our well-being but there's no need for a vast amount of knowledge, expensive plants or acres of lawn. We can grow culinary or medicinal plants and herbs in pots by the front door or along a forgotten side passage, or plant calming lavenders on a windowsill or balcony. In this country we tend to use the front of our houses as a place for cars and bins, covering the earth with paving. Think about what would flourish in your front garden, on your windowsill or grass verge, and if you want to grow tomatoes and that's the sunniest spot, then give it a go. It might even spark some new friendships – when people garden at the front of their homes it encourages neighbourly conversations and interactions. These casual relationships help to boost happiness levels and reduce feelings of loneliness and isolation.

When people garden at the front of their homes it encourages neighbourly conversations and interactions.

Gardening together

Those who have little or no outside space of their own have many alternative ways to get their hands in the earth. Depending on where you live and time demands, there are allotments, community gardens and volunteering opportunities, or it could be as simple as offering to help an elderly neighbour keep on top of their own garden. Sharing gardening or growing tips, cuttings or home-grown produce provides many people with the nature and social fix that is so important for our physical and mental well-being. 'Soil is a great connector,' says human ecologist Zoë Laureen Palmer. 'Without good care for it we have no community.'

Green prescriptions have been shown to reduce pressure on health and social care systems and improve mental health outcomes.

Many people find gardening and growing away from their homes in an allotment or shared space enjoyable because of the change of scene and company, as well as having physical space in which to grow. The combination of physical activity, being outside and close to nature, social connection and the sense of achievement from learning and cultivating forms the basis of Social Therapeutic Horticulture (STH). The charity Thrive has been providing STH for over 40 years and

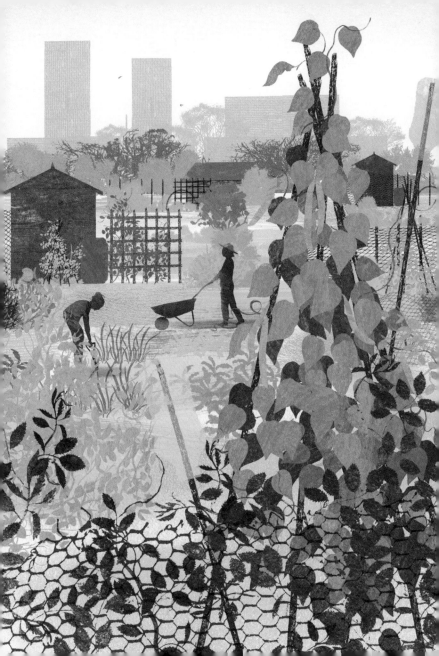

defines it as 'the process of using plants and gardens to help improve physical and mental health'. Gardening projects led by horticultural therapists provide support to people recovering from illness and with disabilities or health needs. The charity also offers short courses and training in STH for people who want to further their skills and support others, either as a practitioner or in a voluntary role. The benefits experienced on both sides make for a very convincing case for green social prescribing, a government initiative to help support people with mental ill health by putting them in contact with community groups offering nature-based activities. Launched in 2020 in the UK, the project has run across seven pilot sites around the country, with the aim of demonstrating the role that nature can play in the treatment of mental health problems. In New Zealand, where green prescriptions have been operating for several decades, they have been shown to reduce pressure on health and social care systems and improve mental health outcomes.

Making a wildlife garden

We can attract wildlife to our outside space in many ways, for example by incorporating bird boxes, hedgehog houses, ponds with insect-friendly plants and flowering shrubs. Creating a wildlife haven can be an enjoyable weekend project and provides a great feeling of satisfaction when the creatures start to visit. Bees and other pollinators need all the help they can get – when choosing plants and shrubs, go for colourful flowers and herbs rich in nectar. Bees favour yellow, purple and blue flowers, and herbs such as basil, thyme, sage, chives and coriander.

Make your own bird seed

Making your own bird seed is super easy. All you need are some seeds (sunflower or nyjer are good), shelled and cracked corn, peanuts (unsalted) and dried fruit such as raisins or cherries. Use a cupful of each ingredient and chop into the same size pieces (about the same as the sunflower seeds).

Add your seed mix to a bird feeder or use it to make fat balls or hanging feeders (great for helping to keep birds nourished through the winter). Just mix your bird seed with melted fat (lard, suet, coconut oil) using one part fat to two parts dry ingredients, mould into shape with your hands and refrigerate overnight before placing outside. And don't forget to add a water bowl, too, unless you have a garden pond.

Coming to our senses

With its huge array of landscapes, plants and wildlife, nature provides us with a unique sensory playground. Practising sensory awareness outdoors will enrich your experience of being in nature and provide a way into mindfulness that many people find easier than sitting indoors and meditating.

Practising sensory awareness outdoors will enrich your experience of being in nature.

Professor Miles Richardson of the University of Derby has pioneered research into nature connectedness and well-being in the UK, and conducted extensive study into what helps us to develop a relationship with the natural world. His team has identified five main pathways that lead to improved connection between people and nature, one of these being 'actively engaging with nature through the different senses'. There are many ways we can do this – to start with you could try choosing a different sense to focus on each time you go out for a walk, and notice how it alters the experience and the things you observe and how you feel. The following pages show some other ways to awaken each of the five senses.

Turn down the noise

Walking and talking together is great and we'll explore this more later in the book. Silent walking, however, is a completely different experience, almost like a walking meditation. Many of us wear headphones while we walk, so even if we're out alone we're listening to music, a podcast or audio book, or maybe talking on the phone. While enjoyable and often time-saving, this is stealing our attention from what's going on around us and drowning out the many sounds of nature. Even if we're walking alone and in silence we can be absorbed in our thoughts and unaware of what's going on around us until we consciously switch on our senses. In her book *The Art of Mindful Birdwatching*, Claire Thompson describes the wonder of tuning into 'nature's radio'. She describes mindful listening as 'experiencing the sounds around us – taking the focus away from labelling what we hear, while bringing our awareness to the features of the sound itself'. It can help if you find somewhere to sit for a while, close your eyes and practise just being present with the sounds you hear.

Change perspective

If you usually walk everywhere, try ringing the changes by riding a bike, for example, or even getting out on the water if you can. And when you're walking, look up rather than down. Hike to the top of a hill. Lie down in the grass and gaze at the clouds. Go the opposite way round a regular loop. Looking up and out has been shown to encourage a more positive frame of mind, whereas looking down can accentuate more negative and unpleasant emotions.

Make a visual memory

Imagine that you're having to describe something and pay attention to the detail: the view from a window; a person you see while you're out walking; a dog that stops to sniff your leg; the bark of the log you're sitting on; the sky when you got up and the sky when you went to bed. Notice how normal things become intriguing if you really study them.

Plant a sensory garden

Any garden is a sensory experience, but there are things you can add to your outside space, specifically with the aim of stimulating the senses. Introducing different sensory elements can help to create a peaceful sanctuary.

- Consider sounds, such as running water or grasses that rustle in the breeze.

- Include scented flowers such as lavender and roses, or herbs such as mint and lemon balm.

- Think about whether you want a space to feel calming or stimulating; pastel shades will be more relaxing and bright colours more energy-giving.

- Grow herbs, lettuce or other edible plants so that you can stimulate your tastebuds.

- Introduce different textures through containers and borders.

Smell the trees

You'll no doubt know some trees by sight, and maybe you touch the bark from time to time, or the branches when you're pruning or harvesting fruit, but you might not be as aware of the smells that all trees emit. The older the forest, the stronger the smell and at certain times of year you'll notice it more than others, and especially after rain. What most of us don't appreciate is that these scents have an important purpose, whether that's attracting pollinators or deterring pests and summoning aid from those pests' predators. Scientists at the University of British Columbia believe that trees may also use scent to communicate with each other about changes in conditions and oncoming predators. In humans, smell is the sense that is often overlooked, and yet it is the only sense with a unique link to the brain's centre for emotion and memory. It is why we like pine trees because they smell of Christmas, and how certain smells such as freshly mown grass can transport us back to a particular moment in time – maybe sports day at school or revising for exams in the summer. Our sense of smell diminishes as we age but if we keep using it we can slow this process. Scent training has been used for people

Spending time in a forest environment has been shown to improve physical health.

who experienced a loss of sense of smell due to Covid-19. A decreased ability to smell has been linked with poor mental health. By awakening and exercising our sense of smell we can train our smell receptors and continue to experience the powerful connection between our emotions and scent. Spending time in a forest environment has also been shown to improve physical health owing to the phytochemicals emitted by trees. Evidence from worldwide studies of the Japanese practice of *shinrin-yoku*, or forest bathing, indicates that observing a forest while engaging the senses leads to an increase in the immune system's NK (natural killer) cells for up to 30 days afterwards. These cells are part of our body's defence against cancer.

Respecting our elders

There are at least 111,000 known ancient and veteran trees in the UK. Unlike ancient trees, veteran trees aren't especially old compared with other trees of the same species but they have ancient features such as wood decay, fungus and exposed dead wood, and a girth that's greater than 3 metres (10 feet). You can find and marvel at our ancient and veteran trees for yourself by checking out the Woodland Trust's inventory and map online. It's thought that there are many, many more than this – up to 2 million, even – and it's possible to add to the inventory yourself if you discover one that isn't already listed. As well as playing a huge role in the

Tree meditation

1. Choose a tree that you can see clearly from a distance and then go over to the tree and find a leaf, seed or any small part of the tree that has fallen to the ground.

2. Holding your piece of tree in your hand, go back to a spot where you can see the whole tree clearly and sit comfortably.

3. Take a couple of slow, deep breaths to set yourself into your space, and then, with your eyes open, focus your mind on the piece of tree you are holding. Notice as much as you can about it, using all of your senses.

4. After a few minutes, look up and focus on the whole tree in front of you. Notice how large and powerful it seems compared with the tiny piece you are holding in your hand. Focus on the tree for a few minutes.

5. Widen your gaze and take in any other trees around you, the sky and everything else. Imagine the universe beyond what you can see.

6. Be at peace with the thought that we are tiny parts of the vast universe, yet made of the same matter and all connected.

ecosystem by storing carbon and regulating water and soil, these ancient and veteran trees provide a habitat for some of our most endangered species and are an important part of our national heritage. Significant trees are protected by the Tree Preservation Order (TPO), which prevents the cutting or pruning of certain trees and areas of woodland, including those on privately owned land, without gaining permission from the local authority. If we lose an ancient tree, it is far from simply a case of replacing old with new.

Tune in to birdsong

Identifying birds' songs and calls takes patience and practice but it is a fantastic exercise in mindfulness because you need to be fully present and in the moment. Returning to the same spot regularly and sitting quietly for a while can help you get to know the birds that visit there and start to tune in to their sounds. Choose somewhere with trees that is relatively low on human traffic and close to some water, if possible. The more carefully you listen, the more you'll start to recognise the different types of call. There's the melodious birdsong usually heard in spring when our feathered friends are giving it their all to attract partners. Companion calls are repetitive sounds that birds use to communicate with one another while they're feeding. A louder, more frenetic and high-pitched call suggests the presence of a predator or a territorial battle between birds. There are plenty of audio guides and apps that help to identify the calls of different birds – it's hard to describe birdsong apart from those birds that are helpfully named after their call, such as the chiffchaff and cuckoo (the male only). You could try recording the chorus on your phone and playing it back to help you pick out the calls of different birds, or when you just need to wind down and relax.

Seek out water

Whether enjoying a holiday in a lakeside cabin or falling asleep to a recording of a waterfall, it's no secret that humans feel calmer in the presence of water. The well-being benefits of 'blue space' are now being compared with those of green space, with studies confirming that spending time by water helps us to relax, improves sleep and encourages us to be more active. While a watery landscape might not always be as easy to come across as a green space, there could be one closer than you think. We've seen an explosion in wild swimming in recent years with people dipping into local bodies of water, from rivers and reservoirs to lakes and, of course, the ocean. Dr Catherine Kelly is a geographer, lecturer, writer and general expert on all matters relating to blue space. She talks emphatically through her own experience of how

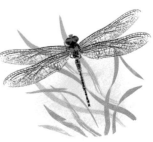

being around water makes us feel happier, more relaxed and playful, as well as benefiting our physical health. When she's not writing or speaking about the links between blue space and well-being, she's witnessing it first-hand at the beach clubs and mindfulness sessions she runs from the seafront in her home town of Brighton. And, naturally, she's no stranger to a dip in the ocean herself, explaining how it always leaves her feeling that 'I can handle my day now'. This mood lift that cold water swimmers experience is caused by 'the stimulating effect of the water on the vagus nerve,' Dr Kelly explains, 'which is what anti-depressants do.'

Swimming outdoors isn't possible for everybody, but we can all benefit from spending time near water. Picnic by a lake in the park, rent a kayak or rowing boat or walk to a waterfall, and on a warm day take off your socks and paddle in a clear stream or along the seashore. A pond or water feature in the garden can help to provide a calming sanctuary for you and for wildlife – somewhere to sit and listen to the soothing trickle of water or watch the visiting dragonflies, butterflies and birds.

Fresh air fitness

When nature provides us with all this space to exercise, you may start to wonder if you need that gym membership after all. Exercise outdoors, and while moving your body and reaping all the physiological benefits, you also get a double wellness boost from being out in nature. Exercise never feels as arduous when you've got trees, plants, water, animals and birds to distract you, and the happy feeling it provides will extend way beyond the time you spend exercising. Consulting agency Gallup has performed a meta-analysis of global studies into the main factors influencing well-being and lists one of their main findings as 'the discovery that exercise is better at eliminating fatigue than prescription drugs'. The same research also revealed that loneliness can double your risk of developing heart disease. A walk, bike ride or jog with a friend might be one of the best things you can do for your health.

Discover your other senses

As well as our five basic senses we have many other 'senses' that guide us. There's spatial awareness, otherwise known as proprioception, and vestibular sense, which controls balance and movement. Then there's a sense of time and direction, a sense that the weather is about to change or that someone or something is approaching us. We talk about a sixth sense as an instinct or hunch, and common sense as something that guides us into making good judgements and behaving in an appropriate way. We rely on these other, less obvious senses to a greater degree when we're out and about, navigating unfamiliar landscapes. Switching off 'autopilot' will enhance the feeling of awareness and connection that you have with your environment.

NATURE CHECKLIST

☐ Switch on your senses. Practise using each of the different senses to notice new things about your surroundings.

☐ Walk mindfully. Leave your headphones and phone and any other distractions in your bag or at home to really engage with your environment.

☐ Get in sync with the natural world by eating seasonally, spending time outdoors in the morning light, winding down in the evenings and allowing yourself periods of rest and recuperation.

☐ Spend time among trees, and bathe in their healing and immune-boosting chemicals.

☐ Get your nails dirty by doing some gardening. You can't get much closer to nature than by plunging your hands into earth.

'The best remedy for those who are afraid, lonely or unhappy is to go outside, somewhere where they can be quite alone with the heavens, nature and God.'

Anne Frank, *The Diary of a Young Girl*

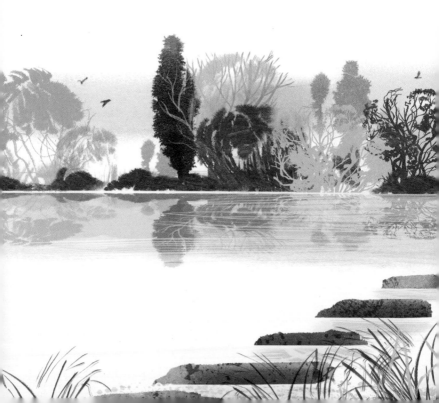

Chapter Two

Nature as Therapy

The effect of nature on mental health is one of the most researched areas of increased nature exposure. In recent years the Covid-19 pandemic offered up a case study in how regular contact with nature helps us to cope with stress, loneliness and anxiety, while providing somewhere calming to relax and interact socially. It's no coincidence that even during the tightest of lockdown restrictions, we were still permitted a daily walk. The experts knew that without exposure to fresh air and nature the fallout could be immense. While it was possible to exercise indoors, talk to people on camera and have most of our basic needs met without really needing to leave the house, it was the local nature reserves, parks and forests that provided a much-needed sanctuary in a time of stress. And new habits have stayed, it seems; in a Wildlife Trust survey 67 per cent of people said they valued nearby nature more now than before the pandemic.

Using nature as a tool for mental well-being is nothing new.

Of course, we may now have more scientific data, but using nature as a tool for mental well-being is nothing new. Gardens have long been a feature of general and psychiatric hospitals, with 19th-century asylums often featuring elaborate gardens as spaces for relaxation and tranquillity, as well as giving an opportunity for engagement in therapeutic outdoor labour. At the Bethlem Royal Hospital in Beckenham, Kent, patients today use the Occupational Therapy Garden for therapeutic horticulture, and the scented plants and textured leaves in the sensory garden provide a gently stimulating and restorative environment.

Gardens in prisons have also been associated with better mental and physical health, with one study showing that having a green view from a cell window led to decreased use of medical services for those prisoners. When horticultural therapy charity Thrive set up a garden in a homeless hostel the service reported less substance abuse. Making good use of the 6,500 hectares (16,000 acres) of land occupied by the NHS is NHS Forest, a scheme launched in 2009 by the Centre for Sustainable Healthcare, which now extends to 330 healthcare sites. An NHS Forest green space might offer a garden for patients and relatives to use as a peaceful sanctuary, a growing patch to provide fresh produce for the hospital kitchen, horticultural experience for volunteers, and woodland and wildflower meadows for nature-based play or outdoor therapeutic sessions. As of 2023 over 100,000 trees had been planted as part of the project.

Scented plants and textured leaves in a sensory garden provide a gently stimulating and restorative environment.

Planting more trees along the streets of our towns and cities can also help to counter the increased risk of mental health problems associated with living in an urban area. A German study looked at the number of street trees throughout the city of Leipzig and concluded that the more trees that people had within a 100-metre (330-foot) space around their home, the less likely they were to be prescribed anti-depressants.

There are many ways in which interacting with nature contributes to good mental health, which we'll explore in this chapter. Of course, mental illness is complex and nature is not a silver bullet or a cure-all. However, it can form an integral part of a care package. And when it comes to maintaining good mental health, nature provides us with a free and accessible tool, with many important life lessons to be learned from simply spending time in and observing the natural world.

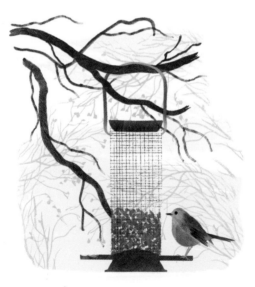

Life lessons from nature

The natural world can teach us many things: slowing down, switching off from our busy lives and taking time to appreciate what is around us has many benefits; practising mindfulness and gratitude in nature can help us to manage our emotions and deal with change and loss; and feeling a connection to and relationship with nature enables us to put our lives into perspective.

Nature is never in a rush

There's a valuable lesson for most of us here as we hurry around from one task to another, rarely taking time to pause and reflect. We're increasingly impatient, seeking instant gratification and comfort. We've lost the ability to be bored; to idle away an afternoon feels wasteful and indulgent. Yet this downtime is part of our natural cycle and is essential for thought processing. Neuroscientists now understand what happens in our brain when we stop and do nothing, and have found that this is when creative and intuitive thinking happens. Rather than filling your time with more stuff to do and rushing to finish so that you can move on to the next thing, allow yourself some time to do nothing and let your mind wander. Often you'll find that your best ideas or solutions spring into your conscious mind when you're daydreaming. Lie down on a rug and look at the sky for a while and see what thoughts arise. Try to be patient and let events in your life take their course as they do in nature. Plant some seeds and observe how, with daily watering and sunlight, they slowly grow into seedlings and then plants producing fruit, vegetables or flowers. Slow down and observe, listen, reflect and ponder. Keep in mind the adage, 'Time you enjoy wasting is never wasted time'.

Slow down and observe, listen, reflect and ponder.

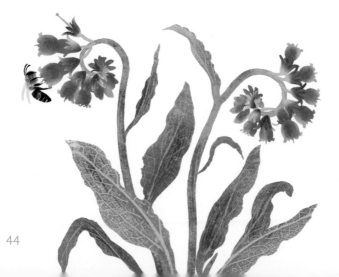

A lesson in mindfulness

Adopting a beginner's mind is one of the key principles of mindfulness. It's about letting go of the preconceptions we gather through experience and life, and allowing ourselves to have an open, empty mind.

- Nature can help us rediscover this beginner's mind when we step back to just observe and listen, without the need to know or be right. Think about how children approach something new, full of curiosity and without expectation.

- Practising mindfulness outside, while walking or sitting somewhere quiet, can be easier than trying to switch off when lying still or sitting down in the home. Next time you set out on a walk you do regularly, try doing it a bit differently.

- Go the other way round the park, take the alternative fork, slow down, stop rushing and pay attention to the details around you. If something catches your eye, pause to look at it more closely. This practice forces us out of autopilot and the habitual way that we all do things, and creates new neural pathways in the brain.

The more you do this, the easier you'll find it to apply a beginner's mindset to other things you do, and you will become more open-minded about new things, people and places.

The importance of switching off

How much better do you feel after an hour out walking in nature than an hour lost down a rabbit hole of social media? Being in nature forces you to look outside of your own life and provides a non-judgemental space to just be yourself. You probably automatically take your phone out with you every time you step out of the house – do you need to? Try leaving it at home if you're only going for a short outing, or, if you really need to take it, keep it in your bag or pocket unless you have something urgent to deal with. It can feel challenging to resist the urge to check your phone but that is a good enough reason in itself to give it a go. The more we resist distraction from our devices, the better we can focus on whatever it is we're doing, whether that is having a conversation or getting some work done. Author and scientist Johann Hari experimented with taking a break from his phone and all social media for three months and writes about the effect this had on his mental well-being in his book *Stolen Focus*. He cites studies of office workers showing that they can only concentrate for three minutes, and

> *The more we resist distraction from our devices, the better we can focus on whatever it is we're doing.*

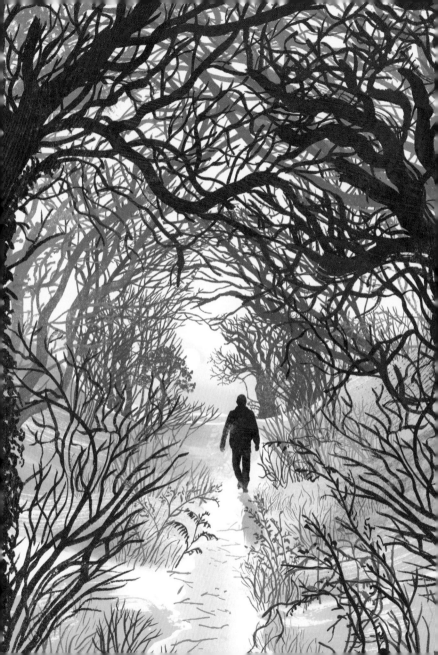

students whose concentration lapses after just 65 seconds, and expresses concern about his own ability to focus. In his device-free time he noticed an unusual feeling of calm quickly coming over him, and an ability to do one thing at a time without distraction. He talks about how his social interactions became pleasing but 'low volume', without a flood of emojis and superlatives, and that he found himself able to focus in 'long effortless stretches' in a way he hadn't since being a teenager. Ditching our devices is not a long-term strategy for most of us, but reducing or resisting distraction is key. If we can silence those pings and dings for a few hours a day while we focus our minds on the present, it can only have a positive effect.

Coping with change and loss

There's no better example of impermanence than nature, with its cycle of life, decay, death, rebirth, restoration and rejuvenation. Observing the changing seasons through the plants, trees and wildlife that surround us, noticing the different shades, sounds and smells as they come and go, helps us to accept that we, like nature, are always in flux. Nature can help us to understand feelings of control and how to let go of them, by relating to things that we live with that are out of our control, such as the weather. During periods of grief many people take solace in nature – knowing that we are part of something bigger can help us to feel held as we process the feelings of fear and loneliness that are often associated with loss. Take comfort in the repetitive, rhythmic cycle of the natural world, knowing that whatever it is that you're experiencing will pass too.

Understanding emotions

Our emotions can sometimes surprise, confuse and even frighten us. Why am I angry or frustrated or sad? What does it say about me? Am I normal? There are many useful meditations that use nature to help us to understand our feelings and thoughts, and how they relate to each other and reality. You can picture your thoughts as leaves or clouds floating along a stream or in the sky. Each leaf or cloud contains a belief or emotion, and you can practise observing these and watching them float away, rather than trying to grasp hold and make sense of each one. Emotions peak and subside like waves and if you remember this it will help you

to ride them out. 'Negative emotions come and go like the clouds but the wide open sky remains,' writes Zen monk and author Haemin Sunim.

Nature helps us to step outside our own heads. After long periods spent living in the wild, writer Gary Ferguson concluded that 'Twenty-five years later I am more convinced than ever that what nature has the power to do is to release us for a time from the tiresome obsession with the self.'

Everything is connected

Sometimes we can feel like a tiny cog in the big wheel of life, and spending time in nature can help to remind us that we're not alone and that everything and everybody is interconnected. Each plant, creature and organism has their role to play and we humans are primal beings, just one small part of the ecosystem. Animals work together in teams to ensure survival. Even plants and trees communicate with one another, and in the forest a mother tree nurtures and feeds the other trees, ensuring that the woodland community thrives. These examples of nature at work not only remind us to respect and care for our natural world but to look out for our fellow humans, and to be caring and generous to those in need, knowing that in nurturing others we are also protecting ourselves.

Plants and trees communicate with one another, and in the forest a mother tree nurtures and feeds the other trees.

How to be grateful

Practising gratitude helps us to feel happier. It encourages better relationships, enables us to cope with adversity and induces positive emotions that impact our thoughts and behaviour. While research into the links between gratitude and well-being is relatively new, the practice is anything but, with gratitude featuring in many ancient philosophies, religions and cultures, from Buddhism to Stoicism. The Roman orator Cicero is said to have called gratitude 'the mother of all feelings'. While you may know of the benefits, it's most likely that you forget to be grateful, or find it difficult or even uncomfortable at times. This is where nature can help. While we might have trouble naming things about ourselves and our lives that we feel grateful for, it's easier to find things in the natural world to appreciate. The morning sun, the sound of the dawn chorus, the rain shower that rejuvenated your lawn, the cowslips painting the meadow yellow. The list can go on and on. And showing gratitude to nature in this way has been shown to have greater well-being benefits than general gratitude journalling. In a five-day study conducted by Professor Miles Richardson, one group was asked to write down three good things they had noticed in

If we can open our eyes and ears to the beauty of nature, we'll never be short of things to feel thankful for.

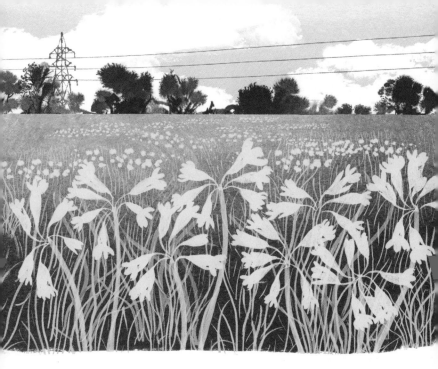

nature each day, another to name anything they felt thankful for, and a control group to write down three factual things. The group that named the nature-related things reported the greatest positive well-being outcomes up to six weeks after the study. Professor Richardson concluded that the findings were due to the increased nature connectedness that people recording things about nature experienced. If we can open our eyes and ears to the beauty of nature, we'll never be short of things to feel thankful for and will feel more a part of the natural world that we inhabit.

The gifts that nature keeps giving

Being out in nature can provide a great variety of benefits: from increased energy and levels of vitamin D, to acting as a natural painkiller; as an antidote to loneliness and the source of endless moments of wonder.

A happiness boost

How good does it feel to close your eyes and feel the warmth of the sun on your face? Sunlight triggers the release of serotonin in the brain, making you feel instantly calmer, happier and more focused. Over a longer period, sun exposure has been shown to help alleviate symptoms of depression and anxiety. We need sunlight to produce vitamin D – experts say that between 10 and 30 minutes of midday sunlight each day is optimum. Low levels of vitamin D are associated with muscle and bone weakness, tiredness, low mood and depression. A lack of sunlight can also disrupt sleep levels and cause low energy levels during our darker months – as many as one in three people experience symptoms relating to the changing of seasons and Seasonal Affective Disorder (SAD), a type of depression that is triggered by a lack of daylight and affects around 2 million people in the UK. Getting out into the sunshine whenever you can, even for a short burst, will help to boost your vitamin D levels, lift your mood and maintain a regular sleep/wake cycle. Being close to water further boosts the effect of sunlight on your mood because light reflects off the water and increases your exposure to the sun's ultraviolet radiation (it's also the reason you're more likely to burn, so always wear sunscreen on a warm day if you're going to be out for more than 15 minutes).

A reliable friend

'Nature is the only thing in life that never disappoints,' writes Gary Ferguson in his book *The Eight Master Lessons of Nature*. The natural world is a constant and reassuring presence, inspiring joy and wonder, comfort and calm at all stages of life. In a fast-changing and uncertain world it can be reassuring to see the first snowdrops burst through the ground in early spring, new buds appearing on the trees, and the changing colours and falling leaves of autumn. Sensory gardens often feature in care homes for patients with Alzheimer's disease, the smells and sensations of plants and flowers tapping into fond memories of seasons gone by. Just like an old and much-loved friend, we need to care for and treasure our natural world.

A mental analgesic

Nature can provide the psychological equivalent of popping a painkiller for a headache. If you're feeling anxious, try this technique commonly used by therapists to engage the five senses and quickly induce calm. You can do this anywhere, but if you practise it in the outdoors, the connection with nature you'll feel afterwards will be extra calming.

The '5, 4, 3, 2, 1' technique

Start by taking a few long, slow breaths, focusing on the exhale.

5. SEE Notice five things that you can see around you.

4. TOUCH Find four things to touch. Try to vary the textures: perhaps a petal, piece of bark, metal fence or blade of grass.

3. HEAR Acknowledge three different sounds; for example, water trickling, a dog barking or leaves rustling.

2. SMELL Find two different scents. This can be the most challenging, but the outdoors should provide plenty of options, from earthy moss to freshly cut grass.

1. TASTE Is there something around you that you could taste? A leaf of pungent wild garlic, perhaps, or a sweet blackberry?

Finish the exercise with another two long breaths and notice how you feel afterwards.

An easier way to talk

Walking therapy offers an alternative to sitting in a room, with the natural environment helping to induce feelings of calm. Talking side by side rather than sitting face to face can also encourage people to feel more relaxed and open. Various studies have shown that walking can significantly reduce symptoms of depression, and that walking in a natural environment is more restorative than taking other physical exercise or simply observing nature. One study from the University of Illinois measured the concentration of children with attention deficit hyperactivity disorder (ADHD) following a walk in a city park, and found that after 20 minutes their attention performance was significantly increased.

Various studies have shown that walking can significantly reduce symptoms of depression.

Outdoor therapy doesn't have to involve walking and it can take place in any outdoor setting – gardening, forest skills and craft can all provide a natural backdrop for different types of therapy. Of course, you can walk and talk with a friend too, and many of us do this without even thinking about why we choose to. As well as the restorative effect of being in nature, the movement and sense of freedom you get from being in an outdoor space means that you're more likely to talk freely.

A grounding influence

As we've heard, the simple act of placing our feet on the ground while walking has a stabilising effect on our emotions. So does lying down on the ground, taking our shoes off, touching the earth or leaning with our back against a tree. This contact with nature and the ground helps to regulate our moods, bringing calmness when we're anxious or energy if we're feeling lethargic. Researchers at New Mexico Highlands University found that brisk walking and running increase blood flow to the brain, potentially improving cognitive health and memory as well as physical well-being.

The comfort of creatures

We can't discuss the healing powers of nature without mentioning the animals that inhabit our world alongside us. From the moments we spend observing wildlife in our gardens, parks and woodlands, to the pets many of us choose to share our lives with, animals make us happier, healthier and better humans. When we interact with animals, by feeding, walking, stroking or playing with them, we produce less of the stress hormones cortisol and adrenaline and our blood pressure decreases, making us feel more relaxed and content. Caring for a pet provides a sense of purpose as well as company. If you have a dog, you're also likely to be more active, with dog owners taking on average 2,760 more steps and around 30 minutes more activity per day than those without. Dog walking often leads to social encounters, too, and those little interactions with fellow walkers or admirers of our canine companions can make us feel better.

Pets can also play a key role in therapeutic care. Studies have shown how dogs can help children with attention deficit hyperactivity disorder (ADHD) to focus their attention and that children with autistic spectrum disorder (ASD) feel less anxious after playing with guinea pigs. In equine therapy, interacting with horses – or just spending time in their company with the presence of a therapist – can help people to unpick difficult emotions and express themselves more freely. If you don't own a dog but would like to walk one, you could check out sites such as Borrow My Doggy (borrowmydoggy.com), where dog owners who need help with walking can make contact with local volunteers. Or if you have an animal shelter nearby, there may be volunteering opportunities there, from dog walking to helping look after the pets and keeping their environment clean. Of course, you can also seek out, observe and appreciate the abundant wildlife on your doorstep, which will make you feel calmer and more connected with the natural world.

A cure for loneliness

Loneliness is such a problem that it's been called a modern epidemic. It's an issue for people in later life, but it's also increasingly a concern for the young. According to the BBC's Loneliness Experiment, 40 per cent of young people reported feeling lonely often or very often, compared with 27 per cent of those over 75. The stigma attached to loneliness means that it doesn't get talked about enough or addressed, especially among the young. It's harder to feel lonely when you're outdoors – you're never truly alone and there are no expectations or judgements. Many people find it easier to connect with nature when walking by themselves. Being alone in nature is often described as feeling more like solitude than loneliness, the difference being that solitude is about choosing to be present in one's own company, as opposed to the sense of isolation that accompanies loneliness. Unlike loneliness, solitude is good for us – it can be rejuvenating and healing, and if it's not something you're comfortable with it tends to be easier when out in nature. Research shows that people who can cultivate solitude are generally more resilient and content, and that time spent alone helps to encourage creativity.

> *Being alone in nature is often described as feeling more like solitude than loneliness.*

Nature also provides many opportunities for forging new relationships, through walking or swimming groups, gardening projects and different volunteering opportunities, for example. Bringing people together outside to engage with each other and connect with nature, to exercise, create and socialise, has been shown to lead to reduced stress, faster recovery from illness, better physical well-being in elderly people, and improved mood and positive emotions. A study by the University of California, Berkeley, found that being exposed to nature improves pro-social tendencies, making us feel more agreeable, kind, generous and trusting.

Moments of awe

In his exploration of awe and how and when we are most likely to experience it, professor of psychology and author Dacher Keltner discovered nature to be the third biggest 'wonder of life'. As part of his research he asked people to be specific about what had triggered feelings of awe, and found that they were most likely to name vast displays of nature such as storms, wildfires and winds, night skies, mountains and the ocean: those moments when we feel a sense of being part of something bigger and

Feeling part of a network or ecosystem can offer a powerful antidote to the isolation and loneliness that is epidemic today.

greater than ourselves, which we tend to forget as we become bogged down with the minutiae of our lives. In his book *Awe: The Transformative Power of Everyday Wonder*, Keltner cites a study in which people were shown videos of awe-inducing nature, and how this was shown to reduce activation in the brain's default mode network (DMN) involved in ego, self-criticism and anxiety. This 'vanishing of the self' effect causes a shift from our 'competitive, dog-eat-dog mindset to perceive that we are part of networks of more interdependent, collaborating individuals. Feeling part of a network or ecosystem can offer a powerful antidote to the isolation and loneliness that is epidemic today. Brief moments of awe are as good for your mind and body as anything you might do', he concludes.

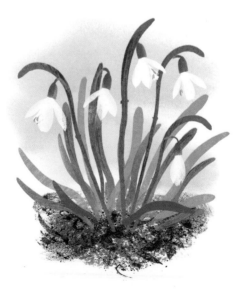

NATURE CHECKLIST

☐ Allow nature to be your friend and your guide, a space where you can be yourself without judgement. Listen to what your mind and body need, and let nature help you find it.

☐ Find awe in the everyday by getting into the habit of noticing small wonders.

☐ Practise gratitude by writing down the things that you notice, and you'll feel more content and connected with nature.

☐ Tap into the healing power of animals – sometimes they understand our needs even better than humans.

☐ Spend time alone in nature and get comfortable with solitude (which is very different from loneliness).

'Nature is not a place to visit. It is home...'

Gary Snyder, poet and environmental activist

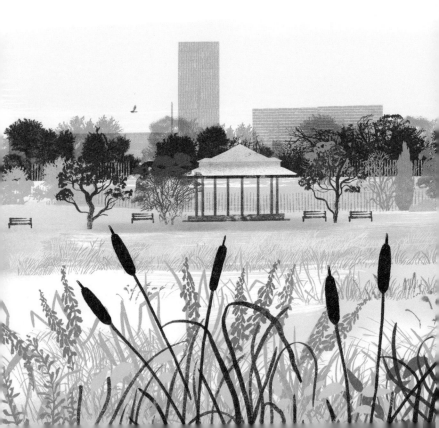

Chapter Three

Urban
Nature

Visit any city on a warm summer's day and you'll notice that every square, park or patch of green is filled with people intuitively grabbing a dose of nature. Eating a sandwich on a park bench while watching the bees pollinate the flowers, or wandering along a city canal beside a pair of paddling ducks, will provide a valuable nature fix in a working day. You don't need to be in the countryside to enjoy nature. It's all around us, and seeking out pockets of natural beauty in the least likely locations can be even more rewarding. If you live in an urban environment (and about 80 per cent of us do), it's even more important that you find time for moments in nature. City life has some benefits, including less loneliness and more accessible health care, but mental health disorders are more prevalent in cities. Proximity to nature is linked to better mental health, concentration, immune resilience and even life expectancy.

Trees, shrubs and plants do much more for our cities than making them look attractive. They absorb pollution, including carbon monoxide, ammonia and sulphur dioxide, through their leaves, bark and roots, and have a significant cooling effect as well as providing crucial habitats for wildlife. Fallen leaves and fruits form mulches that absorb and filter rainwater, helping to prevent flooding and supplying other plants and rivers with clean water. As our cities become more densely populated, the presence of trees becomes even more important. We're seeing ever higher temperatures being reached in summer heatwaves, and with climate change it is expected that these extremes of temperature will become more frequent and intense. Urban trees, and especially those with thick, wide canopies, help to cool down our cities by releasing water vapour (a process called evapotranspiration), reflecting solar radiation, storing less energy than buildings and providing shade cover for buildings and people. According to the Woodland Trust we should be aiming for a minimum of 30 per cent tree canopy cover in urban centres, but in some places there is as little as 3 per cent, and across the country the average is 16 per cent.

While urban greenery makes cities healthier and more pleasant places to live, one UNICEF study found that green spaces can also reduce levels of crime, and improve concentration and school performance among children. When people feel more connected with nature it encourages them to appreciate it and care for it more, so they might think twice about dropping litter or lighting a barbecue in a park or field.

The important thing to remember is that while you might not be able to step out of your front door onto an open field, beach or quiet country lane, the benefits of being outdoors and in nature are just as important. Wherever you live, you can pop on some trainers and go for a walk – University of Leicester researchers found that even 10 minutes of brisk walking daily can yield an extra 16 years of healthy living. Explore your area, wander off your usual routes, and you'll be sure to find some hidden enclaves of nature and wildlife that you didn't even realise were there.

Hidden treasures

Beyond the office blocks and shopping centres, our cities are far from the concrete jungles we might imagine and support a wide range of different habitats, plants and wildlife.

Wonderful waterways

Finding a watery spot in an urban environment can bring an injection of 'blue health' benefits to city life. Studies show that being close to water releases feel-good hormones, making us feel calm yet energised, and that you don't need to be by the coast to experience this. Many of our towns and cities have rivers or canals running through them, and their banks and towpaths make great places for cycling and walking. The dual habitat of land and water provides plenty of opportunities for wildlife spotting, from herons and hedgehogs to water voles and nesting birds. For a different perspective, try getting on to the water on a kayak, paddle board or canal boat, and drift slowly and quietly down the corridors of green, observing life from the water. Pause to watch and listen to anything that catches your attention. Canals move slowly in the nicest possible way and can be a refreshing antidote to the fast pace of city life.

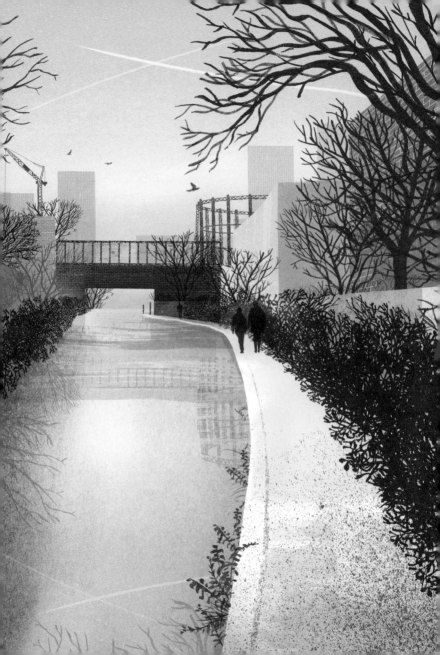

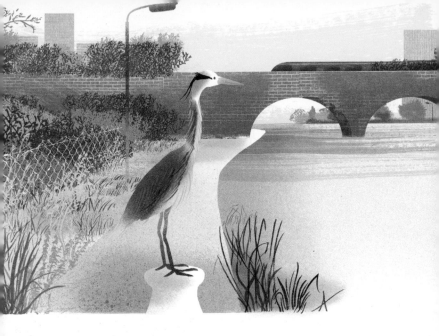

Nature reserves

There are hundreds of nature reserves across the UK – quiet spaces often found in and around our towns and cities that provide wonderful habitats for wildlife. Owned by local authorities but often maintained by local conservation groups and wildlife trusts, a Local Nature Reserve (LNR) exists to protect the biodiversity of an area and also provide a green sanctuary for its human inhabitants. Each will house a variety of different species unique to the area and environment, and you can often download a guide with suggested routes and what to look out for from their website. You can find the nearest LNRs to you via Natural Resources Wales, Natural England, NatureScot and NI Direct. Hunt out one of the smaller, lesser-known nature reserves and you could find that you have the place to yourself. Many have lakes and rivers with reed beds teeming with life, from newts and toads to wetland birds and water rats. They are often great places to spot unusual birds, butterflies and plants – if you're lucky you could find a rare orchid or catch a glimpse of a kingfisher. Observing wildlife makes us feel more connected with the natural world, reduces stress and leaves us feeling calmer and more focused. While we might be tempted to jump on the train and head to the coast on a sunny weekend, staying closer to home and exploring a local nature reserve will often result in a more peaceful and restorative experience.

Churchyards and cemeteries

When you wander through the gates of a churchyard or cemetery you will find much more than gravestones. Often found in the middle of bustling urban environments, our large, sprawling burial grounds provide pockets of wildness and a peaceful haven for trees, plants and wildlife to thrive. In a churchyard, the first thing you'll often notice is yew – these trees are considered sacred in different religions and philosophies, are symbolic of life and death, and are shrouded in folklore and superstition. Planted as guardians of the cemetery often many hundreds of years ago and sometimes pre-dating the churches themselves, the trees were thought to ward off evil spirits and keep wandering spirits inside their graves, while poisonous leaves and berries would deter cattle from wandering in. Yews can survive for thousands of years due to their ability to regenerate by growing new roots through the aged hollow centre of the tree. It's estimated that there are over 600 yew trees in churchyards in Britain that are older than the churches they grow alongside. One of the oldest trees in Europe is a grand yew found in St Cynog's churchyard in the Brecon Beacons National Park, thought to be up to 5,000 years old.

Wandering around a cemetery you'll probably notice several other majestic trees, from oak to ash, planted to absorb noise from nearby roads and provide shade and a focus for visitors. In these wild and often rather unkempt cemeteries, you'll also find wild flowers and shrubs humming with bees and moths in the summer months, while mosses and lichens grow abundantly over gravestones. Benches provide a place to sit peacefully for a while, listening out for birds and small mammals such as hedgehogs and dormice. If you think of graveyards as eerie or morbid, try visiting on a sunny day when the butterflies are circling the graves and the blackbirds are singing, and you may have a change of heart.

City parks

Our urban parks are a longstanding testament to the need for green lungs in our densely populated cities. Many city parks were created in the 19th century, as our urban areas started to encroach more and more into surrounding fields, and it was noted that people living in these environments were becoming deprived of nature and its physical and psychological benefits. The big public parks in our cities were designed for leisure and well-being, often featuring lakes, wooded areas, fountains and sculpture. And they still serve that same purpose today, with popular parks hosting a steady stream of visitors who might be playing a game of tennis, sharing a picnic, meeting friends or walking their dogs, for example. Many old trees can also be found in our parks and on public commons. Next time you're resting beneath the branches of a grand old oak, think about all the people who have sat on the same ground before you. How much life has this tree witnessed? Pick a favourite tree in a park or green space near to your home and return to admire it at different times of the year. Notice how it changes through the seasons and how you also move through periods of growth and rejuvenation, rest and recuperation. An English oak will host and feed over 280 species of insect and bird and produce about 25 million acorns in its lifetime, even though it doesn't grow them for the first 40 years!

Our urban parks are a longstanding testament to the need for green lungs in our densely populated cities.

If you live near a city park, get to know its history, and try to make use of the facilities perhaps by booking a tennis court or visiting the café. Keep an eye on notice boards for events and opportunities to help with gardening, clearing up litter, fundraising and more. Using our parks more often will help to preserve and maintain these integral features of city life.

Urban creatures

We share our towns and cities with a host of wonderful creatures and getting to know what's living around you will help you to feel more connected with nature. Keep your eyes peeled for the wildlife on your doorstep and you might encounter one of the following animals.

Pipistrelle bats

Sit out in a city park or garden in the late evening during spring or summer and you may well spot a few bats from a nearby roost flying overhead. These are most likely to be the common pipistrelle bats that roost in buildings and are less affected by the artificial lights in urban areas than other species. Bats prey on insects so if you're close to water or have a pond in your garden that attracts insects you're more likely to get visiting bats. If you think bats might be roosting in your roof, don't panic; they don't build nests or cause any structural damage like rodents. Bats are under threat – half of the species found in the UK appear on the International Union for Conservation

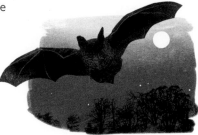

of Nature (IUCN) Red List for Britain's Mammals due to their rarity, rate of decline or lack of data, so creating a bat-friendly environment by turning external lights down or off, encouraging insects into your garden and avoiding the use of pesticides will help to keep numbers from falling further.

Muntjac deer

These relatively small deer (they grow to about the size of a medium dog) are well-adapted to urban environments and can get around quickly and hide more easily than their larger relatives. Introduced to the UK in the 1890s, these deer have thrived, although they're still mainly confined to southern and central England and Wales. They like shrubland and long grass and are pretty good at hiding, so keep your eyes well peeled for those tell-tale ears peeping out from behind a shrub.

Peregrine falcons

While these large, powerful falcons traditionally nested on the edges of cliffs and quarries, peregrine falcons have started to grow in numbers and can be found nesting in tall city structures such as church towers and cathedrals, where they can swoop on and catch their prey in mid-air. Many nesting locations have webcams installed so that viewers can watch the nest and surrounding area at any time of day. Tune in to see the chicks when they hatch, the adult falcons bringing prey back to their young until they leave the nest at about six weeks, and the magnificent sight of the young birds taking their first flight.

Connecting with nature in cities

As well as taking the time to visit all of these green urban places, we can also connect with nature in other ways, such as growing, foraging, swimming and attending outdoor events.

Bring the outside in

Urban living can be made a lot greener with the presence of houseplants. Indoor plants purify the air in our homes by taking in air through the pores in their leaves and stems and removing impurities, from carbon monoxide to dust particles and Volatile Organic Compounds (VOCs) from cleaning sprays, paints and furniture. Cleaner air can help to improve breathing, allergies and headaches, enabling us to sleep better and feel calmer. A few air-purifying houseplants can be a simple yet effective antidote to some of the noise, pollution and stress associated with city life. Just having plants around reminds us of our connection with the natural world, and on days when we don't manage to get

Just having plants around reminds us of our connection with the natural world.

outside for long, looking at and tending to our plants provides valuable contact with nature. Any home, however small, can accommodate a few indoor plants, and if you do your research you can choose varieties with specific benefits, from noise absorption to air purification and sensory stimulation.

Looking at greenery has been proven to reduce stress levels and help us recover from illness more quickly, and the act of caring for something and watching it grow (or at least keeping it alive!) is also good for mental well-being. In a review of studies exploring the link between viewing nature and physiological relaxation and stress recovery, it was found that indoor plants elicit positive health outcomes. While looking at pictures of natural scenes encourages relaxation, it was found that having direct visual contact with real plants (not artificial) was most effective in increasing parasympathetic nervous system (PNS) activity and decreasing sympathetic nervous system activity (SNS), switching off the stress response and inducing feelings of calm. Having plants on or around your desk will have the added benefit of helping you to focus and enjoy your work more. Research by the University of Exeter found that indoor plants can improve concentration, productivity, memory and feelings of job satisfaction.

Houseplants that heal

Peace lily
(*Spathiphyllum wallisii*)
One of the top plants for removing household toxins; its thick leaves can also help with sound absorption.
Needs: indirect sunlight; lightly moist soil.

Bamboo palm
(*Rhapis excelsa*)
A large plant that transpires moisture into the air is a good choice for winter when the central heating is on or in homes where ventilation is poor.
Needs: bright but not direct sunlight; moist, well-drained soil.

Snake plant
(*Sansevieria trifasciata*)
A great plant for the bedroom that acts as a filter, removing toxins from the air during the day and releasing oxygen at night, which will help you breathe more easily while sleeping.
Needs: bright indirect light; well-drained soil.

Golden pothos/devil's ivy
(*Epipremnum aureum*)
One of the most effective indoor air purifiers, this plant has the added bonus of being very hardy.
Needs: medium light; well-drained soil.

Getting growing

You don't need a big garden, or any garden for that matter, to experience the joy and satisfaction of growing your own produce. You can rent an allotment or get creative with different types of containers and whatever outside space you have available. Allotments are great and can provide a peaceful retreat to escape to, but they usually involve a fair amount of time and attention, and it's important to assess honestly what you can afford of both before you commit. Sharing an allotment with a friend, or getting involved in a community garden, can be a good way around the time demands.

City foraging

You might think there are few, if any, foraging opportunities in urban areas, but you'd be mistaken. In city parks and hedgerows and along waterways you can find many edible plants, flowers, fruits and berries. When out foraging we have to switch on all our senses, observing closely the patterns and shapes of the leaves and flowers, feeling the different textures, and enjoying the aroma and taste of our finds. It's a hugely enjoyable, satisfying and addictive activity, and there's a great sense of achievement when you come home from a walk with a bag of hand-picked wild ingredients and then have fun working out what to do with them. Just double- and

Container gardening

When it comes to growing in limited spaces such as balconies, window ledges, patios and roof terraces, choosing what to grow is important. Salad leaves are a good option for window box-sized containers, and if you regularly buy bagged salad from supermarkets, you'll not only be amazed at the difference in taste but also the money you're saving. Add a few edible flowers like nasturtiums and marigolds and you've got a great-looking and -tasting salad whenever you want one. Tomatoes, cucumbers, chillies, peppers, climbing peas, spinach, radishes and spring onions will all do well in smaller containers – just check the variety and size before buying. Whether you want to eat more healthily, save money, support the environment, meet people or just find a fulfilling hobby, growing your own food can provide all of this and more. If you run out of space you can ask if you could place containers in a neighbour's outside space or find a community project to help with. For more ideas on how to green up your city, turn to Chapter Four, Nature Activism.

triple-check your foraged finds
with an expert or guidebook,
make sure you are not
picking from private land
(or seek the landowner's
permission) and avoid eating
wild plants while pregnant
or breastfeeding.

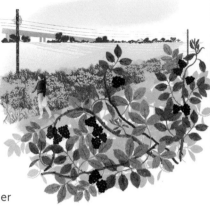

When foraging in urban
environments we need to consider
pollution from traffic, so it's best
to avoid plants growing at the side of
busy roads, for example. Also, be mindful of where dogs
might go to the toilet in parks and on grass verges and tree
beds. Discovering little hidden pockets of plenty is the city
forager's secret – think towpaths, back alleys, streams and
parks. As well as wild plants you can find herbs such as bay
and rosemary, fruits from sloes to figs, and nut trees bearing
walnuts and hazelnuts in public orchards and gardens.
You might also find mulberry trees, which produce large,
blackberry-like fruits in late summer. Keep the foragers' code
in mind: always pick for personal consumption, leaving at
least half of what you find, and remember that foraging is not
permitted at National Nature Reserves (NNRs) and Sites of
Special Scientific Interest (SSSIs).

Six edible urban plants

Chickweed (*Stellaria media*) Grows all year but best foraged from late winter to early spring. Found in gardens, parks and roadside verges, chickweed has a white flower and single line of hairs down the stem. It grows in cooler weather and in large patches. It's a very nutritious green that can be added to salads, pesto and smoothies, and also makes a gentle soothing salve for skin rashes and bites.

Common nettle (*Urtica dioica*) Best picked in early to mid-spring when tender. One of the most ubiquitous yet nutritious plants, its leaves when dried contain up to 42 per cent protein (spinach, for comparison, contains 11 per cent). Nettle has numerous health benefits, from treating urinary tract infections to helping improve allergies and skin disorders. Pick the tender tips of the plant (using thick gloves) and submerge them in just-boiled water for about a minute to take away the sting. You can use nettles in soups, bread and pesto or dry them for tea.

—*continued overleaf*

—continued

Six edible urban plants

Flowering currant (*Ribes sanguineum*) Flowers in early spring; berries late summer to autumn. A shrub often found planted in public parks and gardens. The dark pink flowers taste fruity and can be used in salads or to add flavour and colour to ice creams, sorbets, jams and syrups. The leaves are also edible and best infused in teas.

Hawthorn (*Crataegus monogyna*) Flowers early to mid-spring; berries in autumn. A common tree found in hedgerows, parks and scrubland, with proven medicinal benefits especially for heart health, regulating circulation, heart rate and blood pressure. The white flowers and leaves can be used in tea and the berries make great ketchup or jelly for cheese. Be careful of the thorns when foraging.

Red clover (*Trifolium pratense*) Flowers late spring to early autumn. Found growing in meadows, parks and grass verges, this pretty plant is widely used medicinally for coughs, skin conditions and for menopausal symptoms. The purple blossom has a sweet taste and looks lovely scattered in a salad or as a garnish. The leaves are also edible.

Yarrow (*Achillea millefolium*) Grows March to November. This common plant with frilly, feather-like leaves, a furry stem and clusters of small white or (rarely) pink flowers in the summer can be found anywhere that grass grows, from fields to roadsides and gardens. The whole plant is edible and it is known for its medicinal benefits. These include blood coagulation (it was used to staunch blood and treat wounds in wars), while its high salicylic acid content helps to reduce fever and inflammation. Yarrow smells of pine needles and has quite a bitter taste, so go easy, perhaps adding a few leaves to a salad or to a healing tea for treating fever.

Always check several sources to ensure that you have identified plants correctly, as some have dangerous lookalikes.

Back garden animals

Living in the city doesn't mean that you can't raise animals. If you have enough suitable outside space, have checked any regulations with your local authority, consulted your neighbours and created a safe, enclosed area, then you're good to go. Options include hens or bees, ducks or fish if you have a pond, or perhaps a rabbit or two. A larger enclosed space with grass can even accommodate a small goat. Caring for animals is good for our mental well-being – these loyal and characterful companions give us purpose and help alleviate anxiety, depression and loneliness. They require us to get outdoors and be more selfless, kind and compassionate. Therapy chickens are used in nursing homes and sheltered accommodation to encourage residents to get outside more and have some fun with these sociable animals. They're also kept in prisons, their day-to-day care providing a job for inmates, while offering a calming and therapeutic influence. Adopting a couple of rescue hens will help to combat the problem of poorly treated battery chickens. To find out more about the different animals and the type of care they require, it can be worth popping along to a nearby city farm and observing the animals, talking to the workers and perhaps seeing if there are any volunteering opportunities.

Caring for animals is good for our mental well-being.

Outdoor events

During summer a lot of the things we do socially can be enjoyed outdoors, from cinema and theatre to live music, meaning that you can simultaneously catch up with friends, have a cultural experience and gain some valuable fresh air and nature exposure. Look out for concerts and festivals in parks and fields, outdoor screenings of new and old favourite films, and weekend food markets and events that pop up in the warmer months. Or just arrange to meet friends in a park, each bring a dish to share and a blanket, and enjoy catching up outside until the light fades. Being outdoors in the evening helps to increase the sleep-inducing hormone melatonin so that, when you do go to bed, you'll nod off more easily and have better quality sleep.

Love a lido

Outdoor swimming pools are having a revival and many of our lidos have been restored to their former glory. New urban pools include Hull's refurbished Albert Avenue Lido and the Cleveland Pools in Bath, adding to existing beauties such as Clifton Lido in Bristol and the swimming lake at Beckenham Place Park in south-east London. The Grade II-listed Lido Ponty in Pontypridd has also been brought back to its former art deco splendour. Swimming in cold water has been shown to alleviate symptoms of depression and strengthen the immune system. Starting in the summer and getting accustomed to the temperature, so that you can keep going

Swimming in cold water has been shown to alleviate symptoms of depression and strengthen the immune system.

through the autumn months, could help stave off symptoms of Seasonal Affective Disorder as well as boosting your natural defences against winter colds and other viruses. Try an early morning swim before the city awakes and start the day feeling rejuvenated, or leave the stress of your day behind with a mellow early evening dip. Some lidos have a hot tub or sauna and many offer spa services, yoga and other exercise classes. If you're in the city in the summer, there's no better way to beat the heat and unwind.

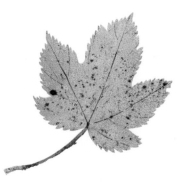

NATURE CHECKLIST

☐ Find the hidden nature spots in your area, from cemeteries to waterways and city farms. Discovering them will open up a whole new natural world.

☐ Slow down so that you can notice what's going on outside. Try walking with a child or dog for a different perspective and to practise the art of pottering, stopping to touch, smell and look at things that alert your senses.

☐ Make your home environment greener by having houseplants around (especially where you work and sleep) and utilising any outdoor space to grow herbs or small varieties of vegetables, or to keep animals.

☐ Spend your free time well by using your local parks and green spaces, walking every day if possible.

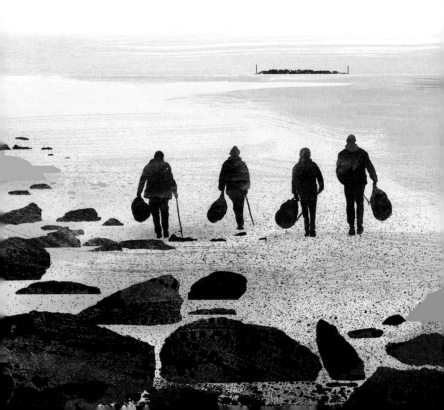

'But man is a part of nature, and his war against nature is inevitably a war against himself.'

Rachel Carson, writer and conservationist

Chapter Four

Nature Activism

When we feel more connected with nature it not only benefits our health, in the many ways we've explored, but it also makes us more inclined to take care of and protect the natural world. As Nick Hayes, co-founder of and campaigner for Right to Roam, says, 'We can't care about something if we're disconnected from it.' So it might just be that the most important challenge we face in terms of the health of our planet and population lies in making sure that everybody has the opportunity to connect with nature, whatever their address, race, age, gender or socio-economic background. If we make nature the preserve of the privileged, and exclude the millions of people living in urban areas where nature is inaccessible or unaffordable to them, then we're making a big mistake.

When people have access to green space, income-related health inequalities are less marked.

Nature activism is about protecting the environment but it's also about making nature, and all its health-giving attributes, accessible to all.

While it might seem that nature is a freely available resource for everyone, that unfortunately isn't the reality. Currently around one in three people in England do not have access to nature near their home and one in eight families has no access to a garden. Many children grow up never learning the names of any flowers or birds or experiencing the joy and freedom of climbing a tree, building a den in a wood or paddling barefoot in a stream. Proximity to nature helps children to concentrate and behave better, and these children will grow into older children and adults that care about the world they live in, and are more likely to adopt pro-environmental behaviours.

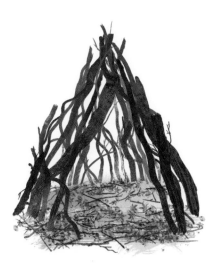

We also know that when people have access to green space where they live, income-related health inequalities are less marked. Professor Rich Mitchell of Glasgow University coined the term 'equigenesis' based on his research into how increasing connection with nature can reduce income-related health inequalities. He found that in low-income areas where people are healthier and more resilient than expected, there is a common contributing factor – they live near parks and woodland. He concluded that rates of income-related mortality were much lower in areas with more green space, and in a further study of 34 European countries he found that access to nature reduced socio-economic inequality in mental well-being by 40 per cent. Green space is considered equigenic because it appears to improve health equality between those with higher and lower incomes. A study by the Environment Agency estimates that the NHS in England could save £2.1 billion every year in treatment costs if everyone had access to good-quality green space.

There are campaigns to extend access rights to our countryside. Currently in England and Wales the public has legal access to around 8 per cent of the hills, moors and coastline and 3 per cent of inland rivers. In Scotland, since 2003 as part of the Land Reform (Scotland) Act, the public has been granted a right to roam, meaning that they can access most land and inland water for recreational purposes, with limitations to protect private property (it doesn't apply to gardens or land with buildings or shelters on it or where crops are growing). The Right to Roam campaign is seeking to gain the same freedom-to-roam rights for the people of England and Wales. The same system as Scotland is in place in other countries such as Norway and Sweden, and they haven't experienced the often-feared damage to the environment by walkers or campers or an explosion of litter from picnics and parties, perhaps proving the point that the more we are able to experience nature the more we appreciate and take care of it.

> *The more we are able to experience nature the more we appreciate and take care of it.*

But it's not just about opening up our countryside – people living in urban areas need to be able to access quality nature without having to get in a car or go on a day trip. Says Nick Hayes: 'One of the main objectives of the campaign is to make access to nature easier for those people living in urban areas who can't necessarily afford day trips or weekends away or holiday homes in the countryside. High quality urban parks, community gardens in housing developments and the planting of flowers and trees in our towns and cities can all make a difference.'

It's easy to feel overwhelmed by the different issues that we face relating to the climate crisis and helpless to make a difference. Many of us feel guilty that we're not doing enough and so avoid the subject and may even avoid contact with nature because it makes us feel panicky or ashamed. Eco-anxiety is a real issue – in a recent survey of 10,000 people, 59 per cent of young people aged 16–25 said they feel very worried about climate change and 45 per cent said it affects their daily lives. However, small changes are incremental, and focusing our attention on doing something, even just one thing, counts for a lot. 'The best way to stave off the climatic doom is by doing things,' says environmentalist Jon Burke. 'Getting involved in a local tree planting group, for example, can be a huge solace and

Many of us feel guilty that we're not doing enough.

antidote to anxiety. Engaging with the wider biosphere helps take our minds off the issues, it heals us as people, heals our community and provides the added benefit of climate mitigation and adaption.'

There are many things we can do to help to make our towns and cities greener, from planting new trees and plants and campaigning against plans to destroy existing trees to supporting the nature reserves and city farms that rely on volunteers and visitors for funding. And if we help to make our countryside inclusive for all and treat it with care and respect, then hopefully more and more of us can reap the numerous benefits that nature, in its many different guises, provides.

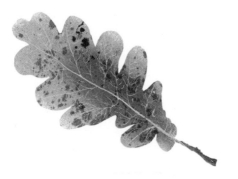

Turning anger into action

The biggest antidote to anger and helplessness is action, and that doesn't have to mean launching a campaign from scratch or making a full-time commitment to your cause. Whether you help to support an existing cause, write an objection to a local planning application you have concerns about, or volunteer a few hours to make your urban park a greener and more pleasant place for people to visit, every little helps. We all have different skills and interests, and harnessing these is often the easiest and most effective way to get started. 'Build on your strengths, do what comes naturally to you and be who you are. Get clear on your motivation and tell the story in a way that's unique to you – knitting or fundraising, scientific research or filmmaking – wherever your talents lie you can make them count by applying them to saving the world,' says Natalie Fee, author of *How to Save the World For Free*. Most of us care about environmental issues, but you're probably interested in one thing more than another. Whether it's animals, children, food or plants, focus on the aspect that you feel most passionately about and think about ways in which you can help. When we play an active role in the shaping of our neighbourhoods we also gain personally from an increased sense of belonging and community. From this, new connections and friendships can evolve, and a feeling of strength gained from the power of action.

Do one thing

When we think about climate change the most common reaction is to focus on what we should stop doing, rather than to think about what we can start to do. For example, we might stop eating meat or stop buying single-use plastic bottles. How about turning that into action by starting to do something helpful as well? If you start supporting local growers and buying more produce from farmers' markets rather than supermarkets you'll be eating healthier foods with fewer food miles and less packaging. Support your local independent shops and restaurants instead of ordering online and you'll help your community to thrive in these tough times. Donate to and buy from charity shops or organise a clothes swap event to help reduce the environmental impact of fast fashion and raise funds. Swapping inertia and inaction for action will make you feel more positive and have a greater impact.

Support your local independent shops and restaurants instead of ordering online.

Plant more flowers and trees

We've heard about all the ways that nature can enhance our sense of well-being, helping us to feel happier and live longer and healthier lives. Some people are making their neighbourhoods greener by planting and growing in public areas – a gentle form of activism that helps people to engage with nature and their community while making the local environment a healthier and more pleasant place in which to live.

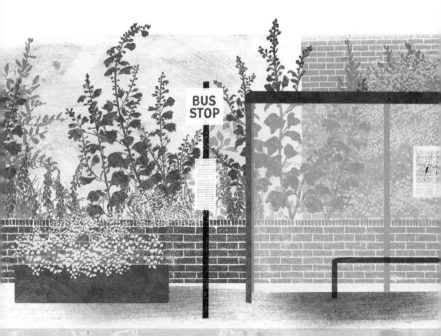

One example of this is the Incredible Edible Network, a group started by some friends in Todmorden, West Yorkshire, who wanted to do something positive for the community and came up with the idea of growing vegetables and fruit in different spaces around their town for residents to help themselves to. There are now more than 100 Incredible Edible groups around the UK busy creating edible playgrounds in schools, planting trees and setting up community gardens. The organisation has launched a campaign to give people the right to grow on public sector land. If you'd like to support the campaign you can write to your local MP asking them to support the Right to Grow Bill – details of how to do this can be found at incredibleedible.org.uk

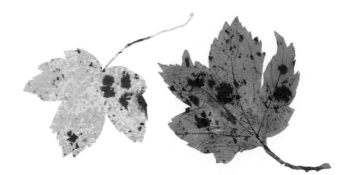

Help to make the countryside inclusive

There are several organisations and individuals working to make the countryside a more inclusive space for all. Here are just a few examples:

Helping young people in London to connect with nature is a priority for Kwesia, aka City Girl in Nature. Growing up in an inner-city area of south-east London, where she says many people feel neglected and marginalised, Kwesia had her life transformed by nature when, as a teenager, she was given the opportunity to take part in a three-week expedition to the Peruvian rainforest with the British Exploring Society. Here, for the first time, she got to immerse herself in nature with 'no phone or judgement' and, on her return, started to think about connecting with young people like herself to see if the beauty of nature could touch them in the way it had touched her. She posts regular videos on her YouTube channel and facilitates walks in the city to help engage young people and show them that nature is all around them and is for them and 'not just white middle-class males in outdoor gear'. Says Kwesia: 'People lose focus on things they don't feel are for them and I just want to use myself as an example and share my love and passion for the outdoors to help everyone get the opportunity to be healed, nourished and live with

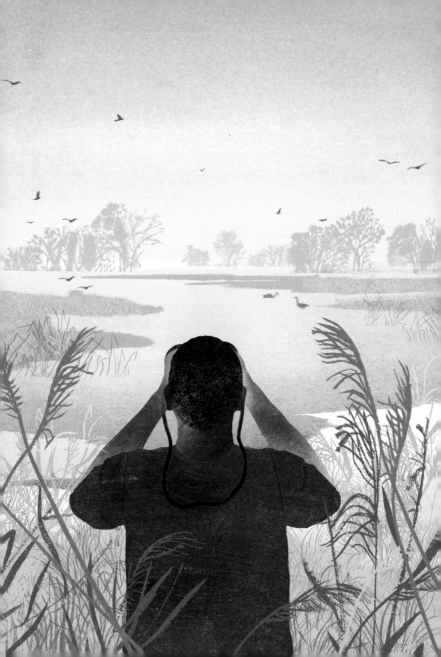

abundance.' She has crowdfunded so that she can help to provide walks, camping trips and talks to connect young people with nature. Listen to her story on the *Nature Bantz* podcast hosted by Hana Sutch, co-founder of the walking app Go Jauntly.

Flock Together (flocktogether.world) is a birdwatching collective to help people of colour rebuild their relationship with nature. The group organises regular birdwatching walks in parks and forests in and around London – no expertise or experience is necessary. Their aim is to expand globally, with 'chapters' already open in New York and Toronto. Founders Ollie Olanipekun and Nadeem Perera say: 'Nature is a universal resource and for too long people of colour have felt marginalised in spaces that should be for everyone.'

Black Girls Hike (bghuk.com) wants the great outdoors to be open and welcoming to all and offers a safe space for women of colour to connect with nature through nationwide group hikes, outdoor activity days and training events.

The British Exploring Society is a charity that takes diverse groups of young people to wild and remote parts of the world, helping to build confidence and resilience and forge relationships. They rely on support from the public, which can be offered in many different ways, so if you're looking to help visit britishexploring.org

Small changes matter

By rethinking some of our everyday habits, behaviours and choices we can all help to be the change we want to see in the world.

Walk, wheel or cycle more

One of the largest contributors to air pollution and ocean microplastics is tyre abrasion. A report by Imperial College London says that 6 million tonnes of tyre-wear particles are released globally each year, while London alone produces 9,000 tonnes of particles from 2.6 million vehicles. While electric cars will help to reduce pollution from fuel, and new regulations on tyre design and manufacturing in the future will help to decrease these plastic particle emissions, it's going to take some time until we're all driving zero-emission vehicles. The simplest way we can help now is by using our cars less and reducing our mileage. If we can walk, wheel or cycle rather than taking the car we'll be helping to reduce pollution in our air and waters, decrease road congestion and danger, and improve our physical health and mental well-being.

Switch off at night

As well as turning lights off inside the house, try to keep any outside lights off or low overnight to help protect local wildlife. Our urban skies glow at night due to light pollution from buildings, cars and outside lighting, all of which affect the behaviour of birds and other animals as well as disturbing our sleep/wake cycle. Insects are attracted to outside lighting and often die on impact, meaning that there are fewer insects as food sources for birds and bats. In the presence of light, bats and owls find it more difficult to hunt, and glow-worms are unable to use their light to attract mates successfully. And it's not just nocturnal animals who become confused – garden birds can be woken by bright security lighting and start singing in the night instead of at dawn. Robins seem to be particularly affected, extending their feeding period into the night.

Turning off the Wi-Fi overnight will reduce electromagnetic radiation in the home (and discourage people from scrolling on phones late into the night!) as well as helping to protect our bees, birds and other wildlife. There have been many studies showing how radiation from mobile phone masts and wireless devices can alter migration behaviour and the nesting and roosting habits of birds – as well as the navigational skills of bees, resulting in lower levels of pollen and honey in hives where the electromagnetic field is strongest.

Save water

Water shortages are becoming increasingly common and we could all save on our water usage. As well as turning off taps, only using the water that you need and using a hosepipe consciously, you could also explore ways to re-use water. Buy a water butt and you can collect rainwater and use it for watering the garden and houseplants, cleaning the car or washing windows. When you live in a country that has plenty of rain, that's a whole lot of free water that hasn't had to go through the expensive treatment that tap water does. As well as rainwater, you can re-use 'greywater' from the bath and bathroom sink to water the grass and plants (not fruit and veg). If you stick to natural bathing and cleaning products, you don't need to worry about adding chemicals to the soil, but all water that contains products or has been used for bathing or handwashing will grow bacteria so should be used within 24 hours. Other ways to conserve water that you might not have considered include buying fewer new clothes and using second-hand or charity shops (growing and dyeing the materials for one T-shirt and pair of jeans can use up to 20,000 litres (4,400 gallons) of water, and clothes are often manufactured in countries with scarce water resources). At home you can fix any leaks or drips, change taps and toilets to more water-efficient models, and keep a bottle of tap water in the fridge so that you don't need to run the tap to get cold water every time you want a drink.

Swap to green or homemade cleaning products

Three inexpensive products that most of us have in our homes – vinegar, lemon and bicarbonate of soda – will do most household cleaning jobs, reducing emissions from Volatile Organic Compounds (VOCs), the chemicals found in many cleaning products, and helping to reduce single-use plastic and save money. A study of roadside air in Los Angeles showed that emissions from perfumes and cleaning products were as much a contributor to air pollution as vehicle emissions. And when you *are* buying products, try to choose eco-friendly versions to reduce the chemicals being released into the environment, and always refill rather than replace where possible.

When choosing 'green' cleaning products it's good to know what you're looking for as some labels can be misleading. Try to choose products free from phosphate, phosphonate and other strong chemicals such as chlorine. Look for biodegradable or recyclable packaging, and a refillable product is always a bonus. Accreditation with the EU Ecolabel or Association for Soaps, Detergents and Maintenance Products (AISE) sustainability stamp will verify a product's green credentials.

Reduce food waste

Buying only the food that you need and using up all the food that you buy is one of the easiest and most effective ways you can help to reduce carbon emissions. Each stage of the journey that food takes, from growing to preparing it in our homes, involves the release of greenhouse gases. And yet we throw away 9.5 million tonnes of food each year in the UK when over 13 million people are struggling to get enough to eat. The situation has improved in the last few years, but we still throw away far too much edible food. The Office for National Statistics estimates that households account for 70 per cent of that waste. According to WRAP (Waste and Resources Action Programme) the average UK household could save £500 a year by cutting food waste, as well as reducing their environmental impact and contributing towards the UK's waste reduction target. Of course, nobody purposefully buys too much food or happily throws food away, but often we get tempted by 2 for 1 deals or bigger 'value' packets and end up with more than we can actually eat before it goes out of date. If you do have surplus food there are apps such as Olio that enable you to swap or give away food in

We throw away 9.5 million tonnes of food each year when over 13 million people are struggling to get enough to eat.

your neighbourhood, and NoWaste that helps you manage the food in your fridge so that you can prioritise what to eat first. If you are buying food on the go, you can also help to prevent food going to waste by registering with apps such as Too Good To Go where cafés, restaurants and bakeries sell 'magic bags' of discounted food that would otherwise be thrown away. Oddbox delivers, direct from farms, fruit and veg that is surplus stock or isn't the right size to make the grade for retail.

Support local farms

If you'd like to buy more locally grown produce you can go direct to the farm by finding your local Community Supported Agriculture (CSA) registered farm. The CSA cooperative supports farmers by cutting out the middleman and providing a direct link to the consumer. There are currently over 150 member farms providing vegetables, dairy, meat, wood and more to local customers in the UK. It's more than just a buy and sell relationship – these community farms rely on their customers getting involved in the production of their food in different ways, from donations and investment to helping with labour. This helps to sustain the farm and provides consumers with a connection to their food and the land on which it's being grown. Each farm is individually run to a common set of guidelines and principles – find your nearest CSA at communitysupportedagriculture.org.uk

Help to clear up your area

Turn a weekend walk into a rubbish-clearing exercise by volunteering to help clear your route of litter. If you're near the coast and fancy a morning at the beach with a purpose, the Marine Conservation Society has details of organised beach cleans around the country. Litter-picking equipment is provided and all ages are welcome – bringing young people along can open their eyes to the waste that ends up in our oceans and washed up on our beaches, as well as the rubbish left by beach-goers every day. There's no better lesson in the importance of reducing waste and leaving no trace than seeing plastic pollution with our own eyes. Trash Free Trails (TFT) is a community of nature lovers and walkers who pick up single-use pollution (TFT prefer this term to 'litter' because it addresses the route of the problem) as they hike, cycle or stroll. An open and welcoming organisation, you can join one of its existing trails or plan and publish your own route and rally the support of the online community. Then it's just a case of getting out there, gathering any rubbish that you find, checking your haul and recycling what you can, and submitting your trail-clean data for the State of the Trails Report at trashfreetrails.org. Their mission is to 'reconnect

Turn a weekend walk into a rubbish-clearing exercise by volunteering to help clear your route of litter.

people with nature through the simple yet meaningful act of removing single-use pollution from wild places'. There are many more locally organised litter-picking walks and events or you could organise your own. A simple exercise like this will not only help to protect wildlife and keep your area cleaner in future (research shows that the less litter there already is, the less likely people are to throw more litter), but will give you a feeling of renewed purpose and positivity.

Keeping our waters clean

Being able to wild swim in the sea or a river, reservoir or lake is one of nature's greatest gifts. While immersing ourselves in cold water works its calming magic on our amygdala, the emotional nerve centre of the brain, we can drink in all the different sensations: the salty smell of the ocean, the vivid shades of green lining the riverbank, a screeching heron, hovering damselflies and that tingling cold feeling as the water hits our skin. No wonder that an outdoor swim never fails to make us feel more alive and invigorated. Yet pollution is plaguing our waters, not only making them unsafe and unpleasant for swimmers but also destroying the ecosystem and wildlife that inhabit them. The issues are complex and political, but we know that far too much untreated sewage is being released into our rivers through sewer overflows and from poor waste management. Agricultural run-off and plastic pollution are other major contributors to ocean and river pollution, meaning that only 14 per cent of our rivers currently meet 'good' ecological status.

You can help the campaign for cleaner waters by supporting the work of Surfers Against Sewage (SAS), perhaps by organising or taking part in a local beach, river or lake clean, or lobbying for greater access to safe spaces to swim. The Rivers Trust has live information on water quality and sewage outflows, and a river quality interactive map that anyone can access via their website: theriverstrust.org

For guidance on how to keep safe while outdoor swimming visit the Outdoor Swimming Society's website: outdoorswimmingsociety.com

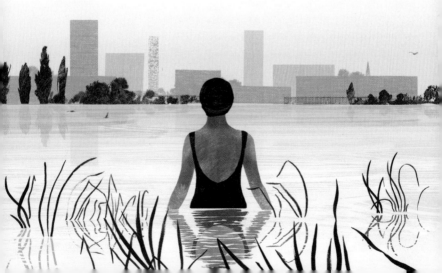

NATURE CHECKLIST

☐ **Be active:** Inaction can enhance feelings of apathy and helplessness whereas any form of positive action will in turn make you feel more positive.

☐ **Be the change you want to see:** Small changes add up and create the possibility for transformation.

☐ **Know your purpose:** Think about what you feel most passionate about and how you can help to protect and preserve this part of nature and why it matters to you.

☐ **Look locally:** Getting involved in a local cause gives you something more tangible to connect with and will help you feel more a part of your community.

☐ **Enjoy the giver's high:** Acts of generosity and kindness also make you feel happier.

'There is no better designer than nature.'

Alexander McQueen, fashion designer

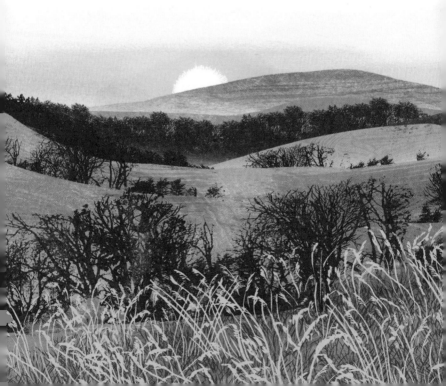

Chapter Five

Nature and Creativity

Nature and creativity are natural companions. When we're out in nature we relax and become freer and more creative with our thoughts and ideas. Using nature as a creative tool encourages us to engage more closely with our environment and derive a different perspective on the natural world. Many of our favourite creative pursuits commonly draw inspiration from nature, from painting to photography, cooking to craft. And research shows that experiencing or creating art triggers brain activity that affects our thoughts, emotions and behaviour positively.

While creativity is about making or creating something new, creative thinking is more about thinking around a problem and coming up with solutions. Both will be enhanced by spending more time in nature. Garry Pratt helps entrepreneurs and innovators access their creative thinking by taking them on outdoor adventures. He writes about it his book *The Creativity Factor*. He says: 'Creativity is something innate in us, it's like play – imagination and creativity are intertwined. Artists visually represent their view of the world, but art is just one outcome of creativity. So is problem-solving and innovation. We are creatures designed to solve problems – it was through creative thinking we navigated the world. Everyone can be creative – we just need to find ways to release it. Going outside and moving in nature is a shortcut to that.'

Most of us have an ongoing tug of war with technology that pulls us away from the natural world into an online world, grabbing our attention and stealing our time. This bombardment of information and stimulation isn't what our brains were designed for, and leads to mental fatigue and a difficulty focusing and coming up with ideas or making decisions. One simple way of countering this is to take a break from technology and spend the time in nature, even if it's just for a few minutes. Attention restoration theory refers to how looking at green and natural scenes rests the pre-frontal cortex of the brain and helps to refocus our minds so that we can think more openly and creatively. In a gently stimulating natural environment, where our attention is given to things such as clouds, birds or trees, we engage in what's known as 'soft fascination' – a less active, involuntary state of attention where the mind can wander, reflect and be creative in thought. This is in contrast to the 'hard fascination' we're engaged in when we're multitasking, stimulating our minds with noise, technology and deadlines, and our bodies with vigorous activity and adrenaline. This soft fascination state helps to restore our mental balance.

Using nature as a creative tool encourages us to engage more closely with our environment.

Observing nature and its cycles can also help us to understand the creative process and be less critical of ourselves. Nature itself is creative and constantly demonstrates all the different ways of surviving and overcoming problems that are available to us. As in nature, there are seasons to our creativity. We too need time to germinate, grow and produce, followed by fallow periods of rest and rejuvenation. Often the expectation is that we spend most or all of our time in the productive stage, but, if we don't take time to find new inspiration and let our minds wander, we soon end up burnt out or stuck in a creative rut.

Creativity is imperfect, like nature. Perfectionism is not natural. A sunset might look perfect today but tomorrow it might be obscured by clouds. A plant may thrive one year and be gone the next. Nature, like life, is unpredictable and often messy. It has dead ends. It has failures. But it never gives up trying. And we can learn a lot from this as we strive to attain perfection. Many of us think we aren't creative because we don't measure up to our standards of what we believe we should be or what we think others are. When you're creating something, it's helpful to remember that the process in itself is useful even if it ends up nowhere. Sometimes you need to try umpteen iterations of something before you find the right one. And even if you end up using the first idea, the process of iterating will not have been a waste of time. Mistakes are useful. If you sow a vegetable seed and it fails, you learn something and

We can also use nature to inspire our own creative process by writing, sketching or creating something inspired by the natural world.

next time you do it differently or try another variety. Most of us are afraid of making mistakes and failing, especially when we're new at something, but unexpected outcomes often lead us down different and interesting paths. Don't beat yourself up if you try something and discover it's not for you.

At times when nature is harder to come by, we can draw on creative resources to get our necessary dose of nature and boost our well-being. The many wonderful works of art, poems, songs, books and documentaries that capture nature's beauty can transport us into a natural environment and soothe our brains and bodies. We can also use nature to inspire our own creative process by writing, sketching or creating something inspired by the natural world, or simply by meditating to the sounds of nature. All of these methods help to shift the nervous system into a restorative state.

By thinking creatively about how to bring nature into our lives we will, in turn, be more creative in all our thoughts and actions.

Where nature and business meet

It might seem like nature is all about leisure and free time, but nature connection feeds into every area of our life and can have a profound impact on the way we think and work. Entrepreneur and walk leader Garry Pratt is passionate about how movement and mindfulness in nature can inspire creative thinking, and has led people on adventures from the hills of the UK to the Atlas Mountains in Morocco. He describes the outdoors as his 'thinking space' and how he came to the realisation that his desk is 'a dangerous place to see the world'. Walking in wild spaces has been proven to generate creative thinking and transform the way people approach problem solving and decision making. Garry says: 'The same bit of your brain that supports learning, memory and cognition is also used for mapping and navigation – by activating that part of your brain in natural settings you can encourage your mind to do things you want it to do creatively.'

If you're struggling to concentrate on your work, a nature-inspired microbreak can help you regain your focus. In one study published in the *Journal of Environmental Psychology*, students were asked to stare at an image of a flowering green roof for just 40 seconds while another group stared at a concrete roof. The green roof group performed better in a test of attention after just 40 seconds, made fewer mistakes and were less distracted. Another study, conducted by neuroscientist David Strayer of the University of Utah, looked at two groups of hikers and found that those who were taking part in a four-day hike performed 47 per cent better on puzzles requiring creativity than those who were waiting to start the hike. These findings are thought to be caused by differences in brain activation when viewing natural scenes.

Garry recommends aiming to spend 20 minutes outside in nature each day (without our phones or other distractions). Something to work towards is his '20:3:3' rule, which includes 20 minutes each day, 3 hours every 2 weeks (on a walk or hike in nature) and 3 days a quarter spent largely immersed in nature. 'Around day three there seems to be massive increase in the brain's ability to process information,' Garry explains. It might be a challenge to do three days every quarter, but it is definitely an aspiration. Ideally you'll spend as much of that time as you can in nature, but you don't need to wild camp or stay in a remote cabin: you can go to a hotel room in the evening as long as the bulk of time is spent in nature.

Enabling creative thinking isn't only beneficial for business; it will impact all areas of life. Garry explains: 'It's increasingly hard to put up walls between work and play, it's all interlinked, it's all part of life and whatever we're thinking about, it's the same process of using creative juices to come up with imagined futures.'

How nature enables creativity

Nature can stimulate and provide inspiration for all forms of creativity, from sketching and journalling to photography, writing and reading. You can also attend creative courses in beautiful surroundings or dance at an outdoor festival. Even social media can be used as a way to celebrate nature, and the ways you interact with the natural world through watching television programmes can increase your knowledge and appreciation.

Nature sounds

The sounds of nature have the power to change the way we think and feel. Experiment for yourself by going outside and listening to the dawn chorus. Tune in to the symphony of blackbirds, robins and starlings. What notes and melodies can you hear? How does it make you feel? Don't worry about trying to name the recording artist: just listen. Studies show that after listening to nature sounds we can think more clearly, and our brains are sharper and quicker. And you don't even need to be *in* nature to appreciate its benefits – if you can't get outdoors, a podcast or recording will do. In one study, led by Stephen Van Hedger of Huron University

College, participants were asked to listen to nature sounds such as crickets and the crashing of the ocean, or urban sounds such as traffic or a busy restaurant, before taking a test. Those who listened to the natural sounds performed significantly better. Try tuning in to the sounds of nature in the early morning before you are bombarded with external noise and stimulation. Taking a greener route to work, playing a nature podcast or spending a few moments tuning in to a recording of the dawn chorus before tackling a challenging piece of work could help you think more clearly and make fewer mistakes.

And now for something completely different ...

ASMR (Autonomous Sensory Meridian Response) is a physical response to certain sounds and causes a pleasant tingling sensation down the spine and goosebumps in some people. Many of the popular trigger sounds are from nature – rainfall, snow crunching underfoot, waves and waterfalls, branches swaying in the breeze. Fans of ASMR say that it helps them to relax, de-stress and fall asleep more easily. There are many audio recordings and videos on YouTube if you want to experiment with the sounds that make you feel the most relaxed.

The joy of a sketchbook

Many people think sketchbooks are the preserve of the artist. A sketchbook is for anyone who wants to express themselves, flex their creative muscles and gain confidence in drawing – and, unlike posting your pictures on social media, nobody ever has to look at it except you. Going for a walk with your book and drawing something that catches your eye is a wonderful way to engage more closely and consciously with nature, and express your creativity in a safe space. With pencil or paintbrush in hand you'll notice more detail than if you were just casually glancing at something as you walk on by, and the concentration it requires will help to stop your mind from ruminating. Drawing regularly will improve your observation skills as well as your drawing skills. Think of it as an exercise in mindfulness and a nature lesson. As artist and environmentalist Nick Hayes says: 'When you are sat drawing, animals relax out of their state of alert, birdsong changes, mammals come out of hiding, you see the world as it is without human intervention.'

oak branch.

Journalling in nature

Another fantastic way to observe and record nature is with a nature journal. Here you can write, doodle, draw, stick and print, inspired by anything you notice in the outdoor world. All you need is a notebook and a pencil – start with something as simple as noting one thing that you see and appreciate in nature each day. Much like the scrapbooks you might have made as a child, you can choose to write a few words, stick in a photo of something you find, doodle or write down a quote about nature, or maybe write a short poem. You can buy journals with prompts for inspiration and there are some beautiful nature journals to admire on Instagram. But don't

Picture this

Are you a visual person who likes to take photos everywhere you go? If so, try to look back regularly at your pictures and reflect on what you've captured and how it makes you feel. You could make a visual gratitude list – aim to photograph something each day that you've enjoyed in nature and file these pictures together so that you can make a photo diary of your observations.

be put off by thinking that you need to produce incredible pieces of artwork or creative writing for it to be worthwhile. The pleasure is in the observing, creating and then the looking back on all the things you've enjoyed and appreciated. You could try doing the same walk each week and noting down the different things you see; by the end of the year you'll have a visual record of the changing seasons to reflect on as well as your own journey. Journalling is a calming practice that, done regularly, has been shown to help reduce stress and anxiety and increase gratitude. Try reflecting on different aspects of nature and how they make you feel depending on your mood that day – expressing your emotions on paper can help with processing difficult feelings and making decisions.

> *Don't be put off by thinking that you need to produce incredible pieces of artwork or creative writing for it to be worthwhile.*

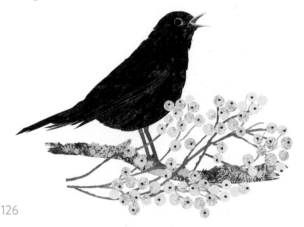

Reading about nature

Losing yourself in someone else's descriptions of nature provides escapism as well as a way of learning more about the natural world. Whether you're keen to further your knowledge of botany or birds, edible plants or urban nature, you can find a piece of nature writing that will be your teacher and guide. If you're visiting somewhere new, reading about the landscape and wildlife where you're going in advance will inspire you to seek out certain experiences on your trip. There has been a recent flurry of nature-inspired memoirs that reflect on the link between nature and emotional well-being, which can deepen our understanding of how nature can help us to heal. Experimenting with various genres or authors will allow you to explore different landscapes and themes, from spirituality and healing to history and social justice.

The wonder of art

If you're feeling stressed, looking at beautiful paintings of natural scenes can have an instant calming effect. A study by British neuroscientist Professor Semir Zeki revealed what happens in the brain when we look at an arresting painting – something many of us will have experienced but not been able to explain. By doing brain scans of individuals while they were being shown paintings by several artists, including many

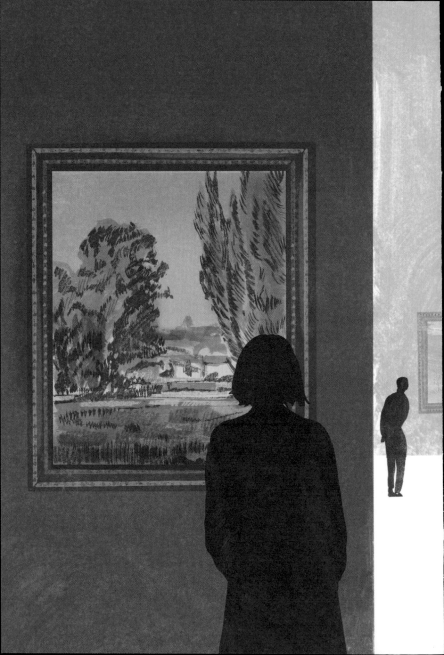

of the great landscape painters such as Monet, Constable and Cézanne, Professor Zeki found immediate activity in the part of the brain relating to pleasure, just like when we look at somebody we love. This study didn't look specifically at reactions to nature scenes, though other research has shown that looking at images of landscapes and seascapes increases dopamine (the pleasure hormone) and reduces levels of cortisol (the stress hormone) in the blood and so decreases health problems associated with chronic stress. In her book *How Art Can Change Your Life*, author and art historian Susie Hodge writes about the emotions that different pieces of art can trigger. Among them are the works of Claude Monet, who painted his famous water lilies over and again to help relieve his depression and anxiety, and to offer others 'an asylum of peaceful meditation'. Many people find his paintings a calming influence just as he once did. In describing the great landscape paintings of J.M.W Turner, Hodge discusses the artist's use of the sun, which features in many of his paintings – including the atmospheric *The Lake of Zug*, which she says captures 'the brilliance of the natural world at dawn giving every viewer a surge of hope for the future'.

If you're feeling stressed, looking at beautiful paintings of natural scenes can have an instant calming effect.

A creative retreat

Signing up to a creative course is a great way to try different skills and maybe kickstart a new hobby. It's no coincidence that many of our creative places are housed in stunning natural environments.

At Dartington Hall Estate in Devon, students can enjoy a huge range of creative experiences with related themes of ecology and social justice. Swimming or kayaking along the River Dart or walking among the estate's ancient trees is all part of the experience. At nearby Sharpham Estate, residents are able to practise meditation and mindfulness exercises in the beautiful grounds, and cook together with produce grown in the walled garden.

West Dean College, in Chichester, Sussex, offers a wide range of creative courses, diplomas and degrees with the backdrop of the rolling South Downs. Students at Newlyn Art School explore the coves and clifftops of West Cornwall for inspiration on many of the school's art courses. Greenwood Days offer courses in traditional wood crafts in the National Forest. The Dreaming is a retreat space in Powys, mid-Wales, with a forest on its doorstep and wild swimming in ponds fed from a waterfall. To find retreats in the UK and beyond visit queenofretreats.com

Be a modern pilgrim

A modern pilgrimage is simply a walk or hike to a special place – it doesn't have to be religious but having a meaningful destination can bring an extra-special element to your walk, helping to make you feel more connected to the land. In the words of the British Pilgrimage Trust, 'Journeying to holy places doesn't imply devout religious intention as holiness can take many forms – cathedrals, rivers, ancient woodland, etc. Holy places are special places toward which you feel summoned to walk.' The journey is relaxed and unhurried, a time to reflect on your inner thoughts and emotions and perhaps connect with others 'while wandering through secret green passages – the bridleways, footpaths, green lanes and hollow tracks of old Britain'.

Dancing in the rain

There's something about dancing out in the elements that feels so fun and free. It's why we love festivals and live music, moving our bodies together under the stars, sharing the energy and letting our hair down with other happy people enjoying a temporary escape from reality. Beyond our teens and twenties, the opportunities to dance the night away often become confined to the odd wedding or milestone birthday. Yet dancing is one of the best forms of exercise for physical and emotional well-being. When we dance, the sensory, motor and pleasure centres of the brain become activated, and when we do it in a natural environment research shows the positive benefits are even greater. With so many festivals to choose from, there's something for every age, musical preference and budget. If you don't want to camp, buy a day ticket to somewhere close to home or where you can stay nearby – or just have some fun in your garden with a few friends and a festival playlist. When life feels all too serious and worrying, letting go of your inhibitions and dancing for a few hours can be just the tonic you need.

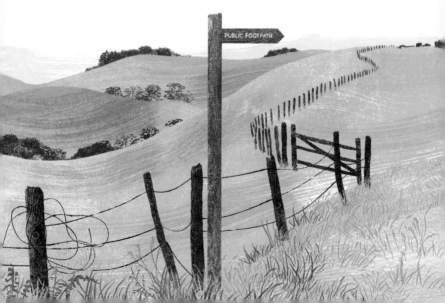

Freshen up your feed

Social media certainly isn't all bad, but it can be a great time thief. Making sure your preferred channels are feeding you information and ideas that make you feel positive and inspired is important, and can have a big impact on how time spent on your phone makes you feel. There are many nature-based Instagram, TikTok and YouTube accounts that can inspire ideas for your own outdoor activities and adventures, from veg growing to foraging walks, nature activities with kids or community events such as beach cleans. Set some time aside to declutter your feeds, unfollowing the accounts that you're not particularly interested in or that don't make you feel happy and adding in more of the kind that fuel your interests rather than your insecurities. Just looking at pictures of green spaces, flowers, wildlife and wild landscapes can provide a mini nature fix when you're stuck inside, while reading about people you relate to and can learn from certainly beats scrolling through endless news feeds.

Watching nature

Wildlife documentaries peaked in popularity during the Covid-19 pandemic, perhaps demonstrating that we find it soothing to look at nature and that we crave the natural world when we're deprived of it. Sir David Attenborough et al not only provide us with a means to observe incredible wildlife in some of the most inaccessible locations, but they also teach us about conservation and bring difficult topics to our attention in a gentle and inclusive format. Several studies have shown that watching nature documentaries actually makes us feel better – perhaps not quite as much as experiencing the real thing, but enough to make it worthwhile and especially as an alternative to other types of programme. In one study, people were shown clips of *Planet Earth II* along with other television programmes, and their emotional responses and stress levels were surveyed. The results showed that after watching the nature programme people scored significantly higher on feelings of awe and happiness, while the news and entertainment programmes increased feelings of fear and anxiety. At the end of a stressful day, choosing to watch a nature programme can be a calming and sleep-inducing way to spend an evening.

NATURE CHECKLIST

☐ Work and play in nature. Nature isn't just for your free time, so why not hold that meeting while walking instead?

☐ Step out of your comfort zone a little to rekindle your creativity. Slow down, draw or write something, take some time out for yourself, walk or sleep in the wild.

☐ Remember that you are creative. We are all born with an innate ability to play, use our imagination and create. We just need to remember how to use it.

☐ Let nature, and not technology, be your distraction. Switch the phone off and leave it in your bag or at home.

☐ Plan your time in nature. Schedule long walks and short breaks that allow you to immerse yourself fully in the outdoors.

Further Reading

Carson, Rachel, *Silent Spring* (Penguin Modern Classics, 2020)

Fee, Natalie, *How to Save the World For Free* (Laurence King Publishing, 2019)

Ferguson, Gary, *Eight Master Lessons of Nature: What Nature Teaches Us about Living Well in the World* (Dutton, 2019)

Hardman, Isabel, *The Natural Health Service: How Nature Can Mend Your Mind* (Atlantic Books, 2020)

Hari, Johann, *Stolen Focus: Why You Can't Pay Attention – And How to Think Deeply Again* (Crown Publishing Group, 2022)

Hodge, Susie, *How Art Can Change Your Life* (Thames and Hudson, 2022)

Jones, Lucy, *Losing Eden: Why Our Minds Need the Wild* (Allen Lane, 2020)

Keltner, Dacher, *Awe: The Transformative Power of Everyday Wonder* (Allen Lane, 2023)

Perera, Nadeem and Olanipekun, Ollie, *Flock Together: Outsiders the Outdoors is Yours* (Gaia, 2022)

Pratt, Garry, *The Creativity Factor: Using the Power of the Outdoors to Spark Successful Innovation* (Bloomsbury Business, 2022)

Richardson, Miles, *Reconnection: Fixing Our Broken Relationship with Nature* (Pelagic Publishing, 2023)

Snyder, Gary, *The Practice of the Wild* (Counterpoint, 2010)

Thompson, Claire, *The Art of Mindful Birdwatching: Reflections on Freedom & Being* (Leaping Hare Press, 2017)

Wohlleben, Peter, *The Hidden Life of Trees: What They Feel, How They Communicate* (Greystone Books, 2016)

Index